Concussion

An Evidence-based Guide to Get You Back From Injury to Your Life

(Step by Step Guide to Concussion Recovery and Diaries to Record Your Experience)

Rodrigo Hunt

Published By **Bella Frost**

Rodrigo Hunt

Concussion: An Evidence-based Guide to Get You Back From Injury to Your Life (Step by Step Guide to Concussion Recovery and Diaries to Record Your Experience)

ISBN 978-1-998038-06-0

Legal & Disclaimer

Table Of Contents

Chapter 1: What Is A Concussion?

Most concussions are not accompanied by a conscious loss. Concussions typically occur as caused by trauma to the brain. This is usually caused by direct contact to the head or an indirect strike on the body. In addition, concussions are typically referred to as a traumatic damage to the brain, in which the symptoms heal on by themselves.

How can we tell if there is the signs of a concussion?

These symptoms are usually a sign of an issue in the brain. It could be nausea, headaches, and problems with intellectual activities that are conscious (thinking thinking, reasoning, recalling and being focused) or emotional reaction (irritability and moodiness) and persistent sleep disturbances or changes in energy levels or appetite. A concussion is regarded as a brain injury. There is no need to get "knocked out" for a concussion to happen In fact, many concussions do not cause losing consciousness. If you've experienced having an "bell rung," it is likely that you've suffered an injury to your head.

The brain is affected in a variety of ways when there is concussions?

Adult brains are a large organ which weighs approximately 3 pounds, and is essentially floating within the skull. It is in a cerebrospinal fluid. It is an absorber of shocks for small collisions. If the brain is made to move swiftly within the skull, concussions are typically the consequence. A straight blow on the forehead or a collision that triggers whiplash-like effects on the body could cause concussion. The force of the impact increases the speed of the head and the brain hits the skull's inner part. The head slows down and ceases to move (whiplash) the brain collides with the opposite side of the skull. A concussion that is a rotational one may occur, where the head quickly rotates across the face from side the other creating strain and shearing in brain tissues. In both cases the delicate neural pathways of the brain may be damaged. leading to sensory or

Neurological problems.

Chapter 2: Signs And Symptoms Of A Concussion

What are some symptoms of concussions?

Some of the symptoms aren't likely appear immediately. These are generally symptoms of early onset and will be described in more depth in the following chapter.

Early Signs:

Uncertain about assignment or the position

* Looks confused or confused.

* Doesn't know what transpired prior to the impact event

* Can't recall what happened following the impact

* Uncertain of game score, game, or opponent

* Makes awkward movements

* Responds to questions slow or does not respond at all

* The person loses conscious (even briefly)

* Displays unusual behavior or changes in personality

The symptoms of a concussion can range from mild to serious and may last for hours, days and even months. If you are experiencing any of the symptoms of a concussion, consult your physician. The symptoms of a concussion fall into four broad categories:

The cognitive process involves thinking, and memory

* Unable to remember or concentrate. Examples include not knowing the date or time or where they are or what they were participating during the time of the injury. Memory loss in the short-term is an indication of concussion. For instance, the patient might ask "Who won the game?" Answer: "We did." Then, "What was the score?" Answer: "21 to 14." After that, he might continue to ask, "Great, who won the game?"

* Disturbance of concentration, such as the inability of focusing on simple items or ideas. It may also be manifested as the inability to follow instructions or react effectively to new information or concepts.

The person who was injured might express a feeling that the pace of life is slowing. Sometimes , a sense of panic can develop or even out of control laughter or crying. If you ask them why the person is usually, "I don't know."

Physical:

* One of the initial symptoms of a concussion typically a mild or severe headache. The person who has been injured often displays an uncomfortable response or sensitive to light. Even sensory input , such as loud noises or the presence of several people talking to the person injured at the same time may cause minor to severe discomfort.

If you can it is crucial to detect any visual impairment. Examine your eyes to see if they are dilation. If the pupils don't react to the light source, it's most likely that you have suffered an injury to the head. If the patient complains of blurred vision or a severe loss of visual in particular if he suffered a blow to the head, see an appointment with a doctor as quickly as you can. Do not move the patient until a doctor or medical specialist has had an chance to evaluate and determine the issue.

Another sign of a problem could include vomiting or nausea. Most often, this problem is not apparent until the injured person is up and moving about for a few minutes.

A lack of or insufficient energy could be a sign of concussion.

Balance issues can affect at a moderate or extreme level, based on the extent associated with the concussion. If someone is injured and has difficulty getting up, raising their arms, walking, or show any other physical impairment, they should be closely monitored.

Emotional:

* Mood could be a sign of concussion. The varying moods of elation and depression could occur abruptly or less quickly dependent on the severity and severity of the concussion.

* A person who has been injured may get easily angry over seemingly insignificant or trivial concerns.

* Nervousness or anxiety that is abnormal.

It is important to consider emotions in the investigation of any type head injury. If the person injured exhibits more or deeper emotional behaviour than usual be sure to keep an eye on the person. The symptoms typically disappear quickly, however being attentive is recommended.

Sleep problems:

• Trouble falling asleep.

* Sleeping longer than usual.

* You're sleeping less than usual.

* Nightmares as well being more tossing and turning than normal.

The concerns with sleep could be complicated, but the most important factor is to remain vigilant and alert to any deviation from the normal. While children show the same symptoms of concussion in adulthood however, there are other aspects that parents must take into consideration in relation to their

child. Here are some of the indicators:

* A persistent headache in which the child continues to complain.

* Changes in diet. As babies grow, moms might notice that her baby isn't feeding in the same way that he typically does. When children are young eating habits, they may vary a bit or even quite a bit.

The way that children play could be affected. Their enthusiasm, or lack of it could suggest that there is a problem.

• Loss of interest in things that they used to enjoy like games, toys or even events that they anticipated.

* Throwing tantrums or becoming angry more quickly or more frequently than usual.

Children who are very young might lose balance faster or lose control of newly learned skills like walking, toilet training etc.

* Consistent sadness.

• Having trouble paying attention. Uncertainty about the severity of an injury requires the intervention by medical professionals.

Chapter 3: Are There Different Grades Of Severity Of Concussions?

There's a lot of debate over the question of whether concussions can be classified into a degree of severity. Almost every concussion is unique to an individual. But certain organizations with expressly certified certification maintain a grade system.

In accordance with the rules of AAN There are three severity levels for concussions.

Grade 1 Concussion:

* Persistent confused; i.e. disorientated or confused.

* There is no loss of consciousness, but mild or severe headache.

* Rapid recovery where symptoms of concussion disappear in under 15 minutes.

Grade 2 Concussion:

* Same is Grade 1. (short-term confusion, but lack of conscious) However, the symptoms of

concussions or cognitive impairments last more than 15 minutes.

Grade 3 Concussion:

* Concussions of the brain at this level typically are defined by any loss of consciousness, whether for a short time (a short amount of time) or longer-term (one minutes or longer).

Many companies are getting more involved in concussion issue. The Mayo clinic provides baseline tests like many hospitals and private companies. Each day we learn every day the most effective and secure methods to handle the issue. If you're the only doubtful about the severity of your concussion, always seek medical attention as quickly as you are able. If you suspect that a concussion has occurred, be sure to follow your doctor's instructions. American Academy of Neurology suggested four step action plan for concussions.

Chapter 4: What To Do If A Concussion Occurs

If you suspect someone is suffering from a concussion related to sports and you suspect that they are suffering from concussions, the AAN suggests a four-step plan of action.

Step 1:

Eliminate the player from the game regardless of whether he or claims they will continue. Examine for signs and signs of a concussion in the event that your athlete has suffered an injury to the body or head. If in doubt you should keep your player off the field. Be aware that many athletes would like to get back into the game and will do anything to be able to return to the game. Don't use scented salts or inhaling stimulants in which they can mask symptoms.

Step 2:

The athlete must be assessed by a medical professional who has years of experience and knowledge in evaluating concussions as well as concussion-related symptoms. Parents, coaches, and spectators should not assess the extent or severity of the injury to their head until they are authorized to perform the evaluation. If no medical professional is readily available, you can make an initial concussion evaluation as described in the chapter 12.

Step 3:

Inform the player's parents or guardians of the possibility of concussion. inform them to talk to an experienced healthcare professional who is skilled in the evaluation of concussions.

Step 4:

The athlete should be kept off the field for the duration of the injury, and until a healthcare specialist, skilled in evaluating concussions says the athlete is not suffering from symptoms and has allowed the athlete to return to playing. A second concussion after the brain has recovered from the initial injury, typically within a brief period of time (hours or days weeks) could slow the recovery, or increase the risk of suffering long-term complications. It is only permissible for the athlete to return to practice or play after the health expert has given the athlete permission to return.

Be aware of this Some experts think that too much inactivity following concussions can be damaging. Pay attention to the signs and symptoms but do not overdo the exercise. Allow the injured person to proceed through the steps being supportive and encouraging them with the assurance that they'll return to their friends and teammates in the near future. Be aware of the signs and symptoms and aware of any deviation that are not typical however, don't overreact.

Chapter 5: Aftercare Of A Concussion

Guidelines for parents, relatives guardians and family members If your child is suffering from concussions, be sure to watch for any of the following signs:

* Looks confused or confused or

* Uncertain with respect to assignments or play

* Uncertain of score, game or opponent

* Reacts awkwardly

* Responds slowly to inquiries.

* Permits loss of awareness (even briefly)

* Displays mood swings , or abnormal behavior patterns.

* Memory is limited of events prior to or after the impact

It is essential to listen to the words your child is saying. In many cases, children explain their symptoms or give an opportunity to demonstrate their symptoms, while being asked to explain the extent to which they feel injured (where and how badly) and what they're thinking about and what they are feeling (emotionally) and what their level of energy could be. Certain things must be considered during the post-concussion time frame to determine whether symptoms persist for hours or days or even weeks. A lot is contingent on specificslike gender, age, normal levels of activity and behavior and any prior concussion history and so on. Every concussion is unique for the patient and their recovery is not the same for everyone.

The protocols should be kept to be kept in the back of your mind. A person's symptoms may be minimal or no symptoms, whereas other suffer from a myriad of symptoms. Although some athletes don't feel any disturbance in their lives following being injured and many experience a decline in their ability to perform academic or other activities (e.g. driving a vehicle) is significantly affected after the concussive event. Any time you experience persisting issues following an injury to the head are a sign to consult medical professionals who are well-trained in the management of concussions. Like most medical issues being treated and diagnosed early, the treatment for concussions are the best option regarding the recovery process and the prevention of further issues.

Training protocols for coaches and trainers

One thing to remember: Don't rush the athlete to play again when he or she has displayed signs of concussion even if the person is your highest-performing player. In addition to the legal concerns, it's simply wrong to do that. Parents have offered you the chance to coach their child and they expect that your main focus is on the health of their child, regardless of the age of the child. As coaches, we're given immense responsibilities within our chosen field. We have to ensure that we're qualified for being able to take on these responsibility. The protection and health of the child is essential.

* Keep in touch with parents and keep an eye for the progress of your child and help them with the post-care procedures even if the athlete is begs for you to "put me in the Coach's office; I'm ready for play. ..."

* Talk to administrators and teachers to ensure that all students are on the same level.

* Offer encouragement , not just to the player, but to grandparents and the other parents.

Keep reviewing your part in the process of recovery knowing that you are an integral element of the decision to allow the person to return to his or her team as well as colleagues.

A note to medical professionals

• You're the primary person to make a decision in this entire process.

* The player can't return to the field without written permission from you.

When it comes to sports often parents, family members and coaches may put an influence on doctors telling them things like, "Doc, I know my player, he's OK. Let me put him back in." Or, "Doc, I know my child. He's going good. He's all set to go. I'm confident." Whatever the advice of others you take the ultimate decision based on your professional training and experience.

* If you're not an "sideline" doctor or medical tech and the patient visits your office to receive treatment The coach and parents will trust your judgement to take the correct choice. In reality caution is essential. It's not always the case, but occasionally doctors do not like a certain sport and may advise children and parents to steer clear of the activity because it's too risky or hazardous. After being a coach for more than 35 years, and having all of my children play various sports, I am able to claim that with the right equipment, coaches diet, and attention sport could be among the most enjoyable experiences one will have. The camaraderie

and fun in loss and winning together, as well as the chance to develop physically, mentally, spiritually and intellectually with your fellow players are all things that no child should be left behind. We hope you're part of the positive process that is greatly appreciated by everyone involved We congratulate you for your efforts. Customize treatment for each patient. Every person reacts differently to concussion.

Chapter 6: Professional's Protocols For Concussion Management

The management of a concussion is requiring the person to take a break and, to some extent restrict physical activity. This is also in the case of thinking processes and the cognitive effort.

* It is recommended to avoid all actions that require an excessive amount of mental stimulation. e.g. texting and spending excessive time in front of a computer and listening to high-pitched music or playing video games etc. Sports Concussion Institute (SCI) an extremely well-respected expert in the field of concussions from athletic events, suggests four key steps for the management of concussions:

1. Awareness and education on concussions

2. Tests for concussions at baseline

3. Comprehensive neuropsychological care

4. Reread the steps covered in Chapter 4.

Concussions can affect people differently which is why a customized method of gradual progression for the person who has been injured returning to sports as well as academics is essential. It is important to make sure we're returning an injury-free, healthy individual to their normal routines including academics and sports.

Always be in the direction of safety.

Chapter 7: When To Seek Medical Attention After Sustaining A Head Injury

Contact a physician If the patient exhibits one of these signs after having suffered a head injury:

* Headaches that get worse

Changes in behavior

* Numbness or weakness in legs or arms

* Difficulty waking up

* Excessive vomiting

* Blood or oral secretions, or fluids

* Changes in the state of consciousness

• Having trouble recognising people, places or names

* More confusion or irritability.

* Speech issues Slurring, stuttering, making mistakes in pronunciation

* Seizures

It is crucial to recognize that it's always a good idea to be in the direction of safety. If an expert medical professional is present during the time of incident, always trust their expertise. A lot of sports require an expert medical professional during their matches, but not always during practices. So, make sure you keep the contact number of the team's nearest physician or EMT to make a an instant access. In addition, many concussions are caused in non-sports-related activities, like falling, playing in car accidents, falling or just life itself. To be secure Keep that number in case in the event of an emergency.

Chapter 8: Protocols For Returning To Play Or Activity

There are four major steps for recovery

Step 1:

* Complete mental and physical rest for a few days until medical approval

There is no school.

• Strictly limited the use of technology

Step 2:

* Resuming school, but with a modified level of involvement

* Maintain limits on technology use

* No heavy backpacks

*No tests, PE, band or chorus

* Keep an eye on any symptoms

* Rest at home

Step 3:

* Continue to follow academic limitations

* Go to school for a full day If you can

* Increase homework and workload

* Check for signs of trouble.

* Relax at home with moderate rest but gradually increase the amount of activities

Step 4:

* Full recovery for academics

* Completely attend school

* Resume normal school routines and tests, homework

* Return to normal activities, including sports scheduling recuperation

Begin through Step 1 . Step 2. Only if an individual has been unaffected for 24 hours. Follow each step only if the person remains symptom free for a period of 24 hours. If the patient is not completely symptom-free at any point then remain at the same stage until he/she is symptom-free.

What to look out for during the days and weeks that follow concussions.

The length of time required to heal from a brain injury that is traumatic could range between a few hours and days, and, in certain instances, weeks, according to gender or age, level of activity or concussion history and other factors personal to the individual. Each individual's brain and injury situation is different, and treatment must be tailored to the specific needs of each person. Although some athletes don't experience a change in their lives following an injury, others experience difficulties to be successful academically and also when they are engaged in other activities for example, driving a vehicle. Any persistent problems after an injury should be an indication to speak with an expert in healthcare who is competent in managing concussions. Similar to most medical conditions the early detection and treatment is the most effective method of recovery and

Prevention of problems in the future. Look out for any changes in your behavior, for example mood swings or outbursts of anger. Activities that in the past provided pleasure can now be annoying or even be resisted completely. In the beginning of healing it is crucial to cut down or eliminate all activities that are necessary like gaming on the computer, texting or any other technical distractions. even listening to music that is loud and other noises, which could hinder healing and cause unintentional harm.

Chapter 9: Concussion Myths And Facts

Myth: You shouldn't take a nap following concussion.

In the event that you are experiencing symptoms currently but they do not get worse and symptoms that are not aggravated are not evident in the initial minutes or hours after concussions, the usual advice is that if the injured person requires sleep it is best to take the time to do so. Sleep is among the most crucial processes that for the brain to begin the process of healing. However, if you notice any new symptoms or symptoms that are already present become worse, it's advised to seek urgent medical attention immediately.

Myth: Any healthcare professional can treat a concussion.

Truth: Sometimes, but not always. It is crucial to ensure that your doctor is familiar with treating concussions and/or neck, head and spinal problems. For more serious injuries like this an experienced specialist may be needed.

Sometimes, this is the specific training offered by neurologists or neuropsychologists.

Myth: The party who is injured is generally aware of the severity of the damage.

The truth is that athletes often aren't aware of the moment they've suffered concussion. They may not be able to acknowledge or admit that they've suffered concussion. Conscientiously, athletes can minimize their symptoms, delaying the extent of the injury or even try to ignore the discomfort. They are eager to play and at times, a self-diagnosis could be the most dangerous decision they make. The self-diagnosis of many times is backed by parents who wish their child to play or by the coach , who considers the player to be in respect and regards the loss of a player as putting the team at risk at risk of being eliminated from the match. If we want to be considered ourselves responsible adults, then we should consider what is the best for the athlete and not be a slave to any individual adult gratification.

Myth: You need to be hit on the head in order to get concussion.

Concussions can be triggered without striking the head directly. For instance, whiplash injuries can happen in the event of an impact to the body , and the neck or head are abruptly jerked back, forward or from side-to-side. The brain's speed is increased in one direction, but it is then decelerated in a different direction, leading to axonal shearing or tearing at the location where the trauma occurred. Other concussion possibilities can occur that occur when the body, and not the head, is shaken or shaken vigorously.

Myth The truth is that it is safe to go back to playing if the symptoms persist but are less severe.

The truth is that experts from all over the globe are of the opinion that athletes shouldn't be allowed to resume exercise until is completely unaffected (showing no signs).

Following a concussion, the brain requires rest and healing time, which isn't possible when it is exposed to physical activities (athletic or not) or cognitive stress (classroom as well as homework) and emotional mood swings that typically occur following an injury. All of these play a crucial part in identifying shifts in behavior in the life of a person. Reintroducing a teenager or child to activities that require physical or cognitive effort prior to the onset of symptoms is a risk for more injury, and may result in a decline in

the performance of the athlete or even worsen debilitating negative long-term effects, such as anxiety, depression and, in certain cases more persistent issues.

Concussion myth: It is only is a problem for the person who has been injured.

Concussions is, like all injuries is able to have significant effects on all those in the influence circle of the athlete that includes parents and families as well as academic staff, coaches and health professionals. However, it is essential to manage concussions with multidisciplinary perspective. Every athlete is able to show the consequences of a concussion at his individual manner. It is important to assess the process of recovery and also to inform one another about the signs, post-care and the reintegration of athletes back into their schooling and routine activities as well as activities. Recognizing these myths and facts is essential to improve our health and wellness to fulfill the obligations given to us. Anybody can sustain concussions, whether either in or out of sport however, prevention is an outcome of education.

Chapter 10: How Do We Prevent Or Reduce The Incidences Of Concussions?

The team sports offer a diverse method of dealing with the issue. Any sport which requires a helmet is the first one to be thought of. According to helmet manufacturers along with the National Operating Committee on Standards for Athletic Equipment (NOCSAE) the purpose of a helmet is to guard against fractures to the skull but not to avoid concussions. It's no surprise that helmets for certain sporting activities are absolutely essential and can reduce the incidence of concussion, however because of the legal environment that manufacturers are barred from using terms like "prevention, reducing, lowers," and so on. in fear of being the subject of ..."lawsuit."

1. Football:

The problems are quite extensive.

* It starts with the company that makes the helmet. In the end, NOCSAE test is an official testing of helmets from junior level to the

professional. After the initial test, many companies require reconditioning of their helmets at least every 2 years. The helmets go to a company that reconditions them in accordance with NOCSAE standards, who put them through various tests to determine if they're safe. When the safety of helmets is found to not be safe, they are taken off the market. When the helmets have been found to be "safe," interior helmet pads and the hardware are replaced while the helmets go back to their organisation.

* The responsibility to keep the helmets in good condition after they are approved is the area of responsibility for the local group. The helmets should be supervised by an equipment manager that works with various teams. The manager of the equipment should be required to attend courses designed to assist him in understanding the particulars of the helmet. Learn more about the dates for these courses by calling NOCSAE or your nearby high school's coach.

* Ensure that all hardware (screws and clamps.) is properly installed.

Make sure that the snaps for the helmet are snug but not too tight. If you tighten the snaps too tightly, it could cause small fractures to the snaps of the helmet and reduce the protection worth for the helmet. These helmets can be costly and require a lot of effort to ensure that personnel who operate the equipment are aware of the duties they are assigned.

Continuous examination of your helmet's condition is an integral part of the procedure. Even the wrong type of paint could make a helmet fail So, only apply the sealer or paint suggested by your manufacturer.

One of the biggest aspects is to make sure that the helmet is properly fitted. Once the participant puts on the helmet the helmet, it must be checked carefully. If the helmet is not snug enough could cause a concussion. If it is too tight, it could result in headaches. Making sure that it fits properly around your head is essential. It can take some extra time to make sure it is right,

However, this type of focus can help to improve prevention strategies.

• Listen to the player. The athlete will tell you if the position is comfortable. Additionally, the level of comfort can change with the seasons. The shape of the body can alter dramatically with significant elevation changes. And, children develop. They get bigger , and the heads of their children grow too. (Sometimes the head of the coach gets bigger , too however, that's another story.)

* The chinstrap can be essential. The majority of players aren't professional and do not want to impress anyone by wearing a chinstrap, or doing it in a way that is not done. The absence of a chinstrap can be considered a violation at every level. The chinstrap must be comfortable but not overly tight.

* In addition to the vast selection of facemasks one important part of the

headgear is the mouthpiece. A lot of organizations offer a standard approved mouthpiece which is sufficient, however for athletes who wear braces or have jaw issues it's best to have an orthodontist or dentist to approve the mouthpiece. A final note on mouthpieces: they are generally made to fit over upper teeth, however studies show that a mouthpiece that safeguards both the lower and upper jaw can produce very favorable outcomes. The majority of rules for youth stipulate that the mouthpiece be attached to the facemask and typically, it's one-piece rubber or vulcanized device.

2. Hockey:

The next step is an extremely lighter Kevlar helmet, which may or might not come with an visor, or perhaps a cage. The manufacturer is essential. We suggest a reputable and approved helmet which has been tested over time. There are many bad helmets on the market, and cost shouldn't be the sole factor when trying to minimize or eliminate the risk of concussion.

These same guidelines for mouthpieces and helmets for football apply to hockey, too. The most significant difference is the chinstrap. The majority of players don't buckle the chinstrap or do not own one. This isn't a great practice for obvious reasons.

3. Cycling:

Particularly competitive cycling, involves many collisions, some at extremely high speed. The helmet for cycling is different. It was designed to provide protection, but must also be aerodynamic so as to provide cyclists the least wind resistance.

The manufacturer is what matters. Be sure to look up the helmet's maker, design and road-tested results. How do they stack up against other manufacturers in the field of concussions?

4. Baseball:

Also , there are cases of concussions. The most common fear young people are afraid of is being struck by a baseball that is thrown by the pitcher. But, more injuries happen during baseball when players slide across a bases, crashing into another player and/or two other players trying play on the field. Batters wear a helmet; fielders do not. In baseball one of the greatest protections against injury is good field communication. The most effective coaches take time with players to go over the their verbal

Signals and on field calls and on field.

5. Mixed martial arts and boxing:

The most significant risk for injuries. In the end, the goal and ultimate success of boxing is to render the opponent unconscious. This is what constitutes concussion. Many of the best boxers from the long, colourful tradition of boxing have suffered severe injuries following their departure from the sport. quit the sport. We often called those "punch-drunk" or "palookas," because they were not able to comprehend interviews or were stuttering in such a way that other boxers had trouble understanding.

Understanding their needs. Certain people have developed diseases such as Parkinson's and ALS or were institutionalized due to the beatings they endured during a fight. Many have died as a result of the punishment they received in the course of fighting. Boxing is a tradition in a number of countries around the globe and it doesn't appear to be likely that it will alter.

Activities that don't require helmets

1. Soccer:

The research is showing that soccer players are more likely to be having concussions. One of the main problems is wearing helmets or not. In the majority of programs, at any level helmets aren't required. However, is this a good thing? Many people think that helmets are not necessary as soccer is one of the "non-contact" sport. However, the 2014

World Cup would suggest otherwise. Many believe that wearing helmets would ruin the look or the essence in the sports. How safe is it?

Of the of the This is an interesting fact: female soccer players are more athletic than men.

There are higher rates of concussions in men than women. The most alarming thing is that a lot of researchers and teachers have noticed memory problems among soccer players in their youth specifically due to "heading" the ball. It is perhaps time to reconsider the necessity of soccer helmets. Speed of soccer balls may be extremely fast and can be hazardous if an athlete tries to alter the trajectory of the ball by using their head.

2. Cheerleading:

Recent studies have placed cheerleading near the top of the list when it comes to concussion. Numerous stunts, a majority of which were previously considered unsuitable due to risks, have now been added to the list.

Cheerleading competition is thrilling. Local regional, state-wide, and even national events have teams of cheerleaders competing against each against each other at a variety of types and levels. A lot of the most successful teams send their cheerleaders to private camps that are run by experienced coaches. These camps can be costly, not to mention the many outfits like kick pants, uniforms shoes, gloves, etc. The problem is that a lot of groups have a greater focus on winning these competitions instead of what is ideal to their cheerleaders. I think that cheerleading is a great sport. The encouragement and support these kids provide to their teams is a great thing. But, safety concerns must be addressed. The complexity and throws of some routines are incredible, but the risk factor needs to be

Not only to youngsters, but also to parents and their coaches, whether professional or amateur.

3. Other Sports:

There are numerous other sports, including skateboarding, basketball as well as wrestling, lacrosse the game of rugby BMX biking, rodeo for kids, water polo , and gymnastics that also require to be taken care of. However it's important to keep in mind that a concussion could happen at work, in play or at school, or any other place where people have the opportunity actively engaged.

Chapter 11: Can We Prevent Concussions From Ever Happening?

Absolutely no! Are we able to decrease the frequency of these incidents? Absolutely! How? Many parents wonder, "How can we get involved with our athlete?" These suggestions offer some ways to do exactly that.

Be aware of the developments in research and equipment. There are many individuals working hard to create equipment that will protect the athlete. There are many devices that can "sense" the potential of concussion through specific devices that are attached to the headband or helmet.

Be aware of what rules apply to the sport. If there are any issues that are not clear modify them.

• Get involved in the organization, if you are not coaching, consider on the board. These organizations cannot exist without honest, dedicated administrative staff who work in the background with little or no recognition and are constantly seeking good people to help out and do their part to make the organization successful.

* Make sure you know your coach. Be sure that the coaches are aware of the things they're doing. Many coaches are wonderful and are committed to their sport. However, sometimes the motivation behind coaching especially at the junior levels, can be questionable. Coaches have said "I'm in it for the kids." What they really mean is "I'm in it for MY kid." They're focussed on living in vicariously the triumphs of their kids rather than on team-building.

To the coaches who have been faithful:

You are the most amazing! Your selfless sacrifice, dedication and your willingness to support your kids are qualities that deserve to be acknowledged and appreciated. The bad things to which I refer to are not directed towards you, the actual coaches, but rather at only a few people who love our sport seriously and turn it into a battle for them. If you're looking to be referred to as "coach" (a profound title) make sure you are qualified. Learn the courses and attend clinics and become educated. As a coach, you must realize that you're an educator, a leader, counselor as well as a guide and often the case, a hero for a young person who requires all of that and more. There is a saying, "I'm only one person, and how can I change the world?" As a coach, you are able to do just that.

You may discover that you are the world to one person. Coaching is a profession. It is the result of every activity you take part in. It begins with integrity, respect morality, sportsmanship character, scholastics and citizenship, and every other good "ism" you can think of. Don't compromise your morals to win on the field that is a result of bending the rules, committing fraud or putting your team at risk.

* Be supportive, not negative. Teams and organizations often fail due to a few of people

do not like the situation, and instead of acting constructively, they turn into the team's official critics. they can cause discord between other parents by attacking coaches in front of their backs and defying anything they don't agree. Take lessons from them and be the opposite.

* Coach training: As coaches are required to study CPR as well as First Aid We must provide certification for concussion awareness and procedures. Certain hospitals and clinics provide courses, however much more must be done to aid coaches with their the certification.

Chapter 12: The On-Field Assessment Guide (The Card)

The Do's and Don'ts of On-field Assessment.

Don'ts

* Do not remove the helmet of the player until a complete assessment is completed. If the patient suffers from neck, head, or spinal injuries, taking off the helmet may have dangerous effects.

* Do not try to lift the person get up to standing or sitting posture until after the test is completed.

* Do not allow crowds to surround the injured person, particularly fans, other players or parents. The worry parents display can cause the injured player to become anxious or be negative.

Do's

When you first approach the injured player, ensure you keep the injured player calm and still. You must ensure that you are in control.

Check if the participant is conscious. In the event that they are not conscious, call 911 for emergency assistance (911). There should be a phone number for an emergency service in case the 911 number is not working or is slow.

If the player is awake, this is the best time to talk. This is also called"the "One second response". Start with the basics, such as, "Where does it hurt?" This is the first chance to evaluate the injury. Ask the injured participant to detail the impact. Does the speech sound slurred, or labored? Does the person be able to respond within a reasonable amount of time to inquiries about the day, timing, the opponent, and so on? Look over in the "symptoms information section" (Chapter 2) in this workbook to determine if the player requires to be taken to a hospital or should it be an injury that is dealt with in the field.

* Absolutely there are no stimulants or odorless salts that trigger a frightened reaction.

Certain tests may be useful in revealing. Ask the participant to put his tongue out and move it left and right, then up and down. This may sound absurd but it can prove very beneficial. Let the participant shift their eyes while following your fingers. Also, observe how fast pupils react to light, or lack of light. So, for example are pupils dilation or focusing? In the evening the lights in the field are sufficient. In the daytime, sunshine or a bright sky are great.

* If the person seems to be responding positivelyto your request, inquire him to sit down. Take your time during this time. Remind the player of this with statements like "Right now, you're the only one we are thinking about, so take all the time you need."

CARD can only be purchased through

"Concussion Awareness Institute Certification Program"

* Request that the participant remove their helmet only if the evaluation was positive.

Don't assist the player to take off the helmet. Allow them to do it on their own. Pay attention to the facial expressions of the participant attentively and ensure that the communication continues. Always ask the player's opinions on any other possible accidents, though the primary concentration should be on the neck, head and the spinal regions.

If you can, let the player leave the field slowly, aiding if needed.

* DO NOT let the injured person unattended in the area.

Before returning to play, the field doctor or medical professional must approve the athlete. If your team are not certified for an on-field injury evaluation the only option is that the player does not return to the field until a medical professional has evaluated the athlete. If there is no one on your team

If you're qualified, my question is "Why not?" There are a variety of courses that are offered by local hospitals and your high school's coaching staff, as well as coaching clinics that have curriculums that include American Red Cross First Aid, CPR instruction, and head trauma training. Remember, you're a coach. Make sure you're the best you can be. this means you need to be educated on much more than simply running games or playing a strong defense. This also means that you are professional. Your character, integrity and ethics are displayed in every practice and in every game. Don't sacrifice. Be fair, but firm. We live in a litigious and litigious society and if you don't want to appear in court one day, you should get certified and follow the rules of on-field medical care. Be aware that any successful treatment for concussions starts long before the injury occurs. It begins with the proper education of athletes parents, coaches as well as athletic trainers, coaches and teachers, as well as others that are in the lives of athletes. Not only does this facilitate the distribution of advanced information to those who are involved in youth sports, it also offers an opportunity for questions to be addressed by experts within the realm of managing concussions.

* It is essential for sports organizations to develop and set up a specific set of guidelines in order to provide certification-based training in the awareness of concussion and protocol. Some clinics and hospitals provide courses, but more is required to aid coaches in getting certified. We can help.

Concussion Awareness: Coach Certification Program

A certification regarding head trauma is vital for trainers, coaches, managers and others. regardless of the the sport's venue.

CERTIFICATION INCLUDES:

* Test on-line

* The On-Field Assessment Guide (THE CARD)

* Certification of Completion

* The Continuing Education Units (CEU coming soon)

* Can include video or audio DVD

Visit our website to find out more details and the start date of Concussion Awareness

Certification   program.
ConcussionAwarenessInstitute.com

Chapter 13: Emerging Technology

Research and Development.

If you search the internet, you'll come across thousands of websites that contain the term "concussion"

on their main pages. More than 95 percent of these sites attempt for you to buy something. Some of the products could be worth your time. It will take some time to find the right one. The biggest issue is that very little is information about concussions. The impact of a head injury to the brain, the signs that follow, recovery and the ability to return to sport, are all topics that have to be dealt with and we tackle this in a number of chapters in this book. There is a great deal of research on the development of more efficient equipment, testing methods as well as a better understanding of the concussion itself. We'd like assurances and assurances from manufacturers of equipment but due to the "lawsuit happy" society and the number of lawyers that must earn a living, no one would want to hear words such as "cure," "reduction," "better," and other such terms. The equipment for sports

Manufacturers know that if a person uses their equipment and suffers injury and suffers injuries, unless they've surrounded their labels with disclaimers they're exposed to serious lawsuits related to risk management. I believe Shakespeare wrote about lawyers as well, and that the Eagles amplified it slightly.

Modifications in the helmet's design like Riddell's Speed Flex which is designed to distribute the force of hits to the head, enhance field of vision , and make internal padding enhancements that reduce the impact from the central point. The new "Sensor" systems measure the amount of impact the body is subjected to after a collision. They transmit the data to the sideline or by using an indicator light to show whether or not the collision is exceeding the parameters recommended by.

A pioneering preliminary study indicates that wearing a specifically made collar may lessen the impact of mild brain injuries or concussion. This research was published online by the Journal of Neurosurgery. Certain helmets have limitations when it comes to stopping certain concussion injuries because of the brain's ability to move inside the skull after impact. This is known as Sloshing, and the fact that it is lessening could be an innovative approach to the prevention of brain injuries. Studies have shown that by blocking Jugular veins using a compressive collar, the amount of blood in the brain was increased to the point that the brain's movement, also known as Sloshing, dramatically reduced. This led to a more than 80% decrease in the torn brain fibers.

Tested on rodents using the standard concussion model in the laboratory. The protection was internal and not outside the human body wearing helmets. Dr. Julian Bailes, Chairman of the Dept. of Neurosurgery and Co-Director of the North Shore University

Health System Neurological Institute as well as one of the principal authors of the study together Dr. Bailes and David Smith, M.D., Joseph Fisher, M.D. They are sure their research is on the proper path in preventing brain injury. The doctor. Bailes explained that the movement of the brain within the cerebral spinal fluid causes the tearing of the fibers that result in a concussion. Rotational motion caused by hitting the sides of the face, head jaw is an important element of the trauma. These and other innovations are the mainstays in solving the concussion issue. Don't compromise your integrity, character or ethics.

Chapter 14: A Word To Coaches

Coaching for more than 35 years...

The landscape of sports has changed dramatically. In the beginning of my coaching career, we would be at the beginning of each day's training and since there were so many kidsthat we would have to knock them with sticks literally speaking. That is not the case anymore. Today, you need to actively recruit at the youth and get involved in every aspect, from fundraising to fundraising (for specific ideas for fundraising and examples, visit our website:

ConcussionAwarenessInstitute.com) getting flyers into schools, car rallies, and so much more. By the way you must also coach. While I was tutoring high school football and youth football simultaneously my wife wanted be aware of what I did to earn an income. The entire youth involvement was unpaid volunteer work. High school coaches provided an fee. After calculating the hours worked in one year and the earnings we earned, we came out to lower than eleven cents per hour. It's funny,

But ask the high school assistant coaches at the high school. Nowadays, kids at school try to be like professional athletes. They spend a lot of their time playing video games that it's awe-inspiring. There was a time when parents wanted their kids to be away from their homes playing sports because they believed that it was healthy and keep them away from TV. One of the biggest changes that have occurred over time is related to the attitudes of parents. I've already talked about the positive impact that parents get, but it is apparent that the majority of parents now consider the video game and television as an excellent babysitter which not only keeps the kids entertained but keeps them away from Mom or Dad's hair.

Let's discuss ethics in coaching...

This advice is applicable to coaches regardless of what sports they coach. I also recommend administrators, teachers, medical professionals, as and parents alike to take a look and gain a bit of understanding of the challenges that coaches have to deal with every day.

The ethics of the ethical coach...

To help promote, refine and enhance the rigors of coaching in order to enhance the performance and development of children as well as young women and men and to coach, inspire and invest in the athletes; to act as examples of integrity and ethical conduct in the realm of competition. To leave aside any personal gain or goals of glory, by putting the needs of these athletes above our own.

Alfred Baden Powell, founder of the Boys Scouts, stated, "Never has a man stood as tall as when he has stooped to help a child." In youth football, coaches for a long time were instructed to put the aside of "adult lust for glory" and instead focus on the advancement of our young to the pleasure of self-confidence and self-esteem. Every youth, high school and colleges, along with their coaches, must be the ambassadors of integrity, ethics and respect for each community that we have an opportunity to be coaches.

Coaching Objectives

* Make this game we love more than an enjoyable experience for children as well as for parents as well as grandparents and friends who play.

Learn to teach winning as an "by-product" of scholastics, civics, sportsmanship, obedience discipline, integrity, and discipline. There are a variety of life lessons to be taught by the sport of sports.

• Understand and teach that sports are games! It's neither the start nor the conclusion of the world. The sun will rise on the next day.

* Become familiar with and equip ourselves with the necessary tools in translating our language we use into a language which can be understood and used by young people. Learn to play the game and an instructor.

Learn to establish an organization for coaches to remove barriers that are in place between local and individual organizations. Join a team of coaches who are determined to become more effective, better efficient, and feel confident about the work they're providing in the world of coaching.

* Learn not just coach, but also teach coaches who are less experienced to ensure that the base of coaching can be boosted.

* Make a promise to not be a reason to join an organization that aims to improve the quality of coaching at all levels.

It is important to win, but not at all cost. Achieving success through honest efforts and with complete integrity is a great feeling. Achieving success without sacrificing morals is an unreal victory.

* After the season comes to an end What will your athlete review you? It is likely that the player enjoyed a successful educational experience , filled more than just games and

memories but also life-changing lessons that will have a positive impact in their lives to come. I've made wonderful relationships with my parents and students alike. They have shaped my life in a variety of ways. I am extremely grateful to my players, and I wish they are feeling the same way about me.

EXPECTATIONS:

What should we expect from coaches? First , there must be communication. It is possible to break down the barriers between rival teams and administrators, teachers as well as parents and fans. and between coaches to understand our individuality. There are often stories of racial conflicts and disagreements between coaches not just between cities that compete, but also within the identical town... And when there is no communication between coaches, these disagreements can escalate into conflicts!.. Sometimes, the motives behind the fights are buried and the conflict persists "just because it's how it is! !" So often when people get the chance to get together and discuss what is they consider important to each of them, we realize that we're very similar to one another. Sometimes , there are remarks made that are misinterpreted or even misquoted by others. These remarks are then taken out of proportion, and are then an argument and cause to declare war, however if they were used in the context of the people affected, the issue would not even be a problem. Coaches are able to meet for friendship or camaraderie, but also to impart training. We are more knowledgeable about the issues and limitations involved in coaching athletes than others.

Most of the time, two youth coaches and a high school coach from the same area don't communicate and have problems, they can arise. It is difficult for an instructor at a high school to comprehend the limitations of a two hour session three times per week, while conducting 2-a-days or watching films during lunch time and early outs for specialist! What is the point of pooling information instead of pooling our ignorance? I don't mean to misunderstand ignorance is simply a ignorance in a particular area. We could conduct internal meetings regarding everything from team management to position coaching, from Scouting for special teams. We can also plan out-of-season events, meet-ups and break bread with friends (eating .... which is one of my favorite things to do). We can develop coaching

procedures for new coaches record the experiences of older coaches; be an inspiration source as a thinking tank for coaches. The idea is to include coaches from different organizations. We coaches could form an organization similar to this and, without doubt, it can fill a void.

There are a couple other issues that I would like to discuss:

1. A Chain of Command When it is possible, we want to keep issues within the teams, however, sometimes it is necessary to establish the chain of command. For coaching

issues each team has their coach's rep, as well as an athletic director. It is our responsibility to talk about issues that require outside involvement. If a coach isn't getting any satisfaction from the coach of his city's

Rep, the coach could make it up in the hierarchy of commands from the athletic director, then the administrator, and follow the steps necessary to resolve these issues.

2. I'd like to speak for an hour on Rule Changes. It happens often throughout the year. I have coaches think of the perfect idea for a rule change , or an idea that could improve the efficiency of things. However, nothing is done. You must record these ideas and then send it to head coaches, then an athletic director. Meet with the referee's representatives and dissect the concepts and, if necessary, present them in a clear manner.

They must be written and submitted them them in writing and submit them to Governing Organization for your sport to consider at the time that is appropriate.

Lastly THE REALITY:

Everyone is aware that there are coaches who take on any challenge to win, regardless of lying, falsifying paperwork or cheating in thousands of ways, illegally recruitment, or abetting the system, and my God why do we do nothing but just watch it happen? Winston Churchill made one of the most powerful remarks in the history of the world in 1939 as Hitler was launching the Holocaust and the genocide of Jews. He stated, (quoting John Locke) "The only thing necessary for evil to abound, is for good people to sit back and do nothing!" It's the time to take an ethical stand in the field of coaching. If something is happening and you are aware of that it's happening, you're not an 'innocent' person when you make a report. You're doing the right thing. The kids are often those who are the ones to pay for an adult who cannot seem to behave in a manner that is honest and ethical.

SUMMARY:

There is a chance to become the type of coach who can make a huge impact on our teams in the years to come if we can find enough people willing to not just make a statement and stand up for their beliefs, but also commit to. There are three types of people that are engaged as coaches... 1. The ones who make it happen 2. those who watch what happens, and third. those who do not know what happened. There's no need to suffer from "Paralysis of Analysis". Get started now. Be part of the solution, not part of the issue.

Chapter 15: What Is The Issue Of "Baseline Testing?"

The Sports Concussion Analytical Tool and Baseline Testing.

I'd like to acknowledge my friend Mr. Lance Townend of Canadian Sports Risk Management for his kind gesture of giving us permission to reprint a portion of the data his company came up with on the subject of test baselines.

One of the biggest discoveries made by the Geneva Conference when the Sports Concussion Analytical Tool was created was the conclusion that it was necessary to establish a Baseline was necessary to be used as a way of comparing in the event that a SCAt test was given. In the present, conclusive results can be achieved. SCAt and the SCAt as well as the SCAt2 tests were created in Geneva Medical Convention in Geneva Medical Convention in

Switzerland. Doctors from around the globe discussed concussions specifically , diagnostics, testing and treatment. Their resulting publication of SCAt as well as the SCAt2 tests has been embraced across professional and amateur sports organizations and associations. SCAt 3, the latest test instrument baseline measurement, offers an examiner the possibility to determine the exact distinction between the pre and post incident.

The main reason for conducting an initial test is to build the foundation of individual data that form an operational matrix of the normal brain function of the person. After this data has been documented, it can be used as an element against which comparison can be made contrasting the normal functioning to the post-injury condition that the brain is in. There are a variety of test programs that are able to be used with this baseline. One of them is BESS (Balance Error Scoring System) that consists of a set of questions that are scored and in comparison to the test that was used as a baseline.

Other systems, such as SWAY Balance is a mobile device that gives a rapid response, which is used in the sideline protocols used to treat concussion. It is a lot of focus being paid to the subject of concussions that massive processes from assessing concussions to the procedures for "Return To Play," are expected to be announced within the next few months.

The Concussion Awareness Certification program, the second level will cover Baseline SCAt3 as well as all the post-concussion tests available. We will be adding new materials when they are available. Check out Chapter 16 in this book.

Chapter 16: Certification And The Website:

ConcussionAwarenessInstitute.com

Sports is now an extremely interesting aspects of our time. There are more sporting events and sports in the present than at any other period in the history of mankind. Sport has also been viewed as controversial, particularly in a time when the media's attention is on the dangers associated with concussions.

In almost every professional or college, high school, and even youth sport there is a requirement that coaches are certified in CPR and First Aid. CPR and that's fantastic. However, when looking at these crucial safety concerns there are a few points to be taken into consideration.

1. First Aid. Sprains, cuts, bruises fractures and so on. These are not necessarily within the realm of sports. They're a part of almost every sport that we participate in. Therefore, it's a great practice to make coaches are

aware of procedures to follow in the event that there is an injury.

2. CPR (Cardio Pulmonary Resuscitation) is crucial as it addresses the possibility of dying. It is the process of restoring the lung and heart function. If someone isn't breathing, we should no longer wait around for medical assistance to come. We must act immediately. That's the reason CPR classes are available

In every community, there is in every community through Fire Dept, hospitals, clinics, and private companies.

First aid is essential and a first-aid kit is vital. How often does it get used? It is often, due to the fact that a lot of things happen. Usually not life threatening....sometimes. CPR...

How often? I hope not often. But in the event that it is necessary organizations have recognized that it is important to be prepared and that means getting certified.

Let's discuss the 800-pound gorilla that is present in this room. CONCUSSIONS! What is the reason there isn't a recognized, standardized training program that is mandatory for trainers, coaches, etc. ?

What are the possibilities for concussion? Every practice and game, every accident,

each fall, every fall and on. Keep in mind a couple of points. First , we aren't doing anything to scare anyone. We are especially not trying to convince them of being too defensive and kicking their children away from sports...ANY sport! The benefits, especially of the team sport, is tremendous. From sportsmanship to team camaraderie, planning morality, honour, and other life experiences ....I could continue. That's why kids don't have to lose out on opportunities due to a lack of knowledge. Also, don't forget...according the study conducted by Chicago Medical and Northwestern University Neurology More than 74 percent of ALL concussions don't result from sports.

Additionally, a recent study of the causes of concussions revealed that riding a bicycle is ten times more likely to cause CONCUSSIONS THAN ATTACKLE

FOOTBALL!! What do you think of Pop Warner Youth Football?

They have made excellent choices regarding their practices and by limiting certain kinds of contact, they've admitted in an article in the Los Angeles Times article that within the last 2 to 3 years , they have experienced 1% or A LOWER incidence of concussions annually!

THE WEBSITE:

In the absence of a comprehensive and professional agenda for certification in concussions, Concussion Awareness Institute is developing a state of the advanced protocol system to certify coaches, trainers and administrators, which includes parents of children who ride bicycles and just about anyone interested in learning exactly what they should do in suspected concussion. We have created an two-tier system, one that is primarily focused on quick "on-field" guideline application and a higher level of advanced sideline protocols, including various R & program for D (BESS, SWAY, and other). The second level will be more extensive than the level one. Both levels will be presented in a modular, timed format. It is important to note that the "CARD" (see Chapter 12) will be only available for those who successfully pass the Level One Certification . The program is comprised of a series of questions on the internet that address all aspects of "on-field" issues to risk management. The focus isn't the way to play or coach football. It is how to avoid getting you or your business legally sued.

In light of the ever-changing nature of our understanding of concussions, the certification is expected to last for two years. Then, the coach or the candidate can be eligible for the "renewal" certification, also available online.

The site will offer not just fundraising ideas as well as a platform that coaches can access and download offenses defenses specific teams, and scouting information and even video outline templates that are adapted to coaching positions, with a variety of camera angles to provide cutting-edge techniques, increasing the capacity to coach your particular sport.

Chapter 17: Case Studies

I'd like to begin this section by stating that the majority of concussions are minor and don't develop into a traumatic condition. But, it is well to inform people that a concussion can be serious problem. Therefore, below are two cases that address the most serious injuries.

Study Study One - Dr. Stephanie Mills: 2014 Ms. America and mom.

A message from the school was received: "Your daughter was knocked out of the gym class. It is imperative that you pick her up as soon as possible." Brooke was an "A" student in the class of freshman. The next morning, she bent down to grab the ball when an unidentified child kicked it. The ball, his foot and her head met in one go and she collapsed into a blackout. After the incident, Brooke's headaches became more severe. As a chiropractor, her mother could provide her frequent adjustments to her spine to ease the pain in her head and to ease fatigue, however, her memory was a problem. Brooke would enter the room without knowing the reason, and she would lose memories of family holidays and was unable to recall what she was instructed in the classes prior to the head trauma that took place. Brooke was afflicted with concussions.

At the beginning, Brooke committed herself to recovery with restorative cognitive exercises not TV, no texting and no school or taking classes. Physical activities stopped, even the dance team. After a week without classes and other activities the pressure to get back was evident. Brooke was not a victim of previous baseline tests for concussions prior to her injury. Doctors were not able to show coaches and teachers that she was able to return to regular activities. As as a parent Doctor. Mills needed to become her daughter's advocate. If the counselor recommended Brooke return to the gym within a few days of her accident her mother resisted. As chiropractor Dr. Mills knew the risk of Secondary Impact Syndrome. A second concussion after the first has healed completely can be even more debilitating and could even be fatal. Brooke was unable to complete her freshman year at school. At the time of this writing her memory, a lot of it remain unreturned. Wearing protective equipment in gym classes might have helped her stay safe from injury. A lot of concussions are not preventable however the most effective solution is to establish routine testing for all middle school and the high school age students. The risk of not getting the diagnosis of a concussion is significantly decreased, and it allows for better monitoring of the process of recovery.

I played fullback during high school andon occasion, I played the football. In one match, I ran well through the middle, but was attacked. My helmet was one-bar suspension (these are no longer used). The moment I fell my facemask hit the ground and my helmet flew away. The safety who might have been preparing to be the punter, punched me squarely on the forehead. According to witnesses, I jumped and was dragged back to the huddle while the other player was taken off the field. The quarterback thought the play was quite excellent, so he called the play again. My team was seated at the line of play. the center snatched the ball, and the quarterback then turned to pass the ball over to me but I was not there. I was back at the point where the huddle was set up looking up at the sky. I'm told I was removed from the field, taken into the medical facility, was discharged after which I returned to home. The game was scheduled for a Thursday night. The next day I awoke at school and set out with the goal of playing football the next day. My coach noticed me in the hallway and asked me what I did. I responded. "Great, we're going to whip Beal Tech today." He was looking at me in a strange way and then asked me "What day is it?" I answered, "Thursday." He told me, "OK, come with me." He took me into his car and took me back to hospital. I was completely lost for the span of 24 hours in my life. I don't have any memory of ever being a part of the game. The memory has gone. This is based on witness stories. I experienced severe headaches for the duration of a week but then I had no problems whatsoever. I was extremely fortunate not to experience any problems however the loss of memory was quite alarming. I've had numerous occasions which I have described as being able to hear the "bell rung," not only due to sports, but also an accident in a car and getting tripped down the flight of steps or a door closing by force against the side of my head and more generally, engaging in what insurance adjusters call "high risk activities." It's LIFE! It is impossible to live our lives in a secluded, secure environment from the possibility of negative consequences that can befall on any person. Our lives can be lived in joy and excitement with the knowledge that what's in the future will be based on more than the actual events but the way we react to them.

Coach and Author Michael (Mike) Shaw Bio

Mike is a native of Canada. He has played in competitive Hockey, Football, Basketball,

Baseball, Volleyball, Track and Field Swimming, Diving and Wrestling, Tennis, Badminton and more. He's always been a close person to sports. He was employed by Sports Productions, Inc., Cleveland, Ohio then began his own company together with the American Basketball Assn. He relocated in to California in 1969 and was married in 1969 to Toni. They had three children: Casey, Stephanie and Cory. He was a football coach during 35 seasons at both the junior level as well as high school. He was a youth coach at Rowland Heights, CA, for 28 years as the head coach with the total of 286 victories and only 33 losses but most importantly the team he was with have won more sportsmanship and academic awards than any other coaching staff across the nation. Over the years, Mike has been the director of some of the best coaching classes in the United States. He was the vice president of the National Football Foundation and Hall of Fame and is the first youth football coach to be selected for the Hall of Fame.

Mike has been involved with The United States Olympic Committee and has written books for other athletes. Mike is currently Chaplain. He runs two companies: Coaching Software Solutions, LLC and CSC Enterprises, LLC a real estate investment company.

Chapter 18: Parents

There is a saying that baseball's the National Pastime, but football is the National Passion. Because of this one of the most important problems facing sports is the public's reaction to the constant media coverage of concussions during sports. Parents are at the forefront in this regard, since they are the ones that must deal in anxiety of concussions that can cause brain disorders, including depression, memory loss or suicide, as well as the death of their children. In addition, due to the raging media coverage of these issues and it's been reported that the National Football League (NFL) as well as the National Collegiate Athletic Association (NCAA) each high school, and each youth football team across the country seem to be losing players. This is right, starting with the young and moving on to college, high school and eventually the professional ranks over time.

over the past five years, over the past five years, there has been a dramatic reduction in participation in sports over the past five years. The estimates suggest that around 50% of children entering ninth grade have experienced some form of concussion and the majority of them didn't realize that they had suffered the injury. A majority of these concussions weren't related with organized sport. Did you realize the odds of children being 10x more likely be injured while playing on bicycles than football?

Children are involved in games with horses, playing pick-up games, and other types of activities unsupervised that could cause injuries. These are cyclones of energy and activity. Think about the number of times that a kid slips or is injured in an accident at home. Concussion is at the top in the minds of coaches, parents and trainers as well as administrators of contact sports. The reality is that virtually every athletic sport, particularly ones that are prone for head or body collisions, impacts, could result in the possibility of a concussion.

But, the increased awareness of concussion is not a cause for end the popularity of sports that involve contact. It should instead be considered as the moment that made youth sports, including sports for kids, safer than ever.

From the NFL and the National Hockey League (NHL) from the NFL and National Hockey League (NHL) to the NCAA and the National Federation of High Schools (NFHS) and even the youth and beginner sports, many changes have been implemented to minimize head contact during exercises. In the case of those in the younger age bracket Kickoffs have also been removed. In addition, the increased awareness has resulted in massive investment, which has resulted in improved equipment and rules changes and protocols that safeguard players. Recent studies have shown that through the use of the USA Football's "Heads Up" education programs and the newly-implemented Pop Warner Football rules against excessive contact, the rate of concussions have decreased.

The awareness campaign has shed information on the other aspects of participation in sports. For instance, the Mayo Clinic recently published a community-based study called "High School Football and Risk of Neurodegeneration." The findings of the study indicate the following: "Football players have no greater risk for dementia than members of chorus, glee club or band, and participation in football is actually a protective factor against depression and suicide."

Studies have also shown that our youngsters became sedentary - if they quit

playing sports like football or other--the negative consequences of such a life-style would be immense with the potential for increasing obesity, hypertension and diabetes among other health risks. However, even the overweight child may see the benefits of reducing cardiovascular risk from playing sports. Like we said earlier the advantages of playing sports in teams are extremely positive. Here are some additional reasons why parents should urge their children to stop spending money playing video games, and to join sportsfor learning lessons in life, camaraderie, playing with other people by setting goals for the whole group and being in a secure and enjoyable educational setting and a sense of accomplishment and many more. My boys played football until when they were seven years old. The people they met then became their most trusted friends for the rest of their lives. When they gather they continue to discuss their childhood and high school years. In football, the players were taught to live life with enthusiasm, enjoy the pleasure of conquering challenges and recognize that success does not only come about winning games, but equally a result of the hard job of practicing. They were able to apply the wisdom they gained from the game in a way and use it for other activities. For a more in depth coverage of the fears associated with concussions including the latest research and statistics refer to our concussionAwarenessInstitute.com website.

I'd like to thank the Dr. Uzma Samadani for her contributions to the content in Chapter 18. A short biography follows, and a more complete biography is on the ConcussionAwarenessInstitute.com website.

Uzma Samadani MD PhD is an expert in neurosurgery who is also a researcher in brain injuries at Hennepin

County Medical Center, the largest Level One trauma center in Minnesota and among the most busy in the nation.

Affiliations:

* Rockswold Kaplan Endowed Chair for Traumatic Brain Injury at Hennepin County Medical Center.

* Associate Professor of Neurosurgery at the University of Minnesota.

* Neurosurgeon attending in the Minneapolis Veterans Administration Medical Center.

* Executive Committee of the American Association of Neurological

Surgeons/Congress of Neurological Surgeons Joint Section on Neurotrauma and Critical Care.

* Chair of the Scientific Program for their conference in collaboration in conjunction with National Neurotrauma Society.

• Liaison with the Board of ThinkFirst Foundation, a brain injury prevention group.

*She has written over 40 peer-reviewed scientific articles.

*Dr. Samadani also serves as an unaffiliated neurotrauma specialist with the National Football League.

Chapter 19: Minimal And Brain Trauma

This isn't a book about brain traumas that are severe or the often debilitating physical disabilities caused by these injuries. It is the story of an essentially invisible disease.

Research indicates that 75%-90 percent of all traumatic cerebrovascular injuries involve concussions, or any other type of MTBI (mild traumatic brain injury. This type of neurological injury that is frequently ignored or dismissed even by those who is suffering from the injury.

What is the media's coverage of Brain Injury

Since 2002, conflict that have raged in Iraq as well as Afghanistan have put the issue of traumatic brain injuries in the news media's spotlight. This was especially true following the time that ABC News anchorman Bob Woodruff was lost to a bomb on the road in Taji, Iraq in 2006.

In a remarkable recovery mostly a reflection of what doctors from the military on the field had to learn firsthand regarding treating brain injuries Woodruff returned for work 13 months later.

Woodruff's life began with a medically-induced insanity. He underwent nine surgeries to remove a portion of his skull as well as reduce the pressure over his skull.

While his physical capabilities returned at an incredible pace but his recovery in cognitive terms was a gruelling process. Seven years after his recovery, Woodruff is still struggling with difficulties in speaking as well as vision loss in the top quart on both eyelids, as well as hearing loss.

Woodruff's recuperation, and the recovery the recovery of Arizona Congresswoman Gabrielle Giffords who was killed by a gunman in Tucson in 2011 are both dramatic and inspirational. However, results like those suffered by Andrew Blackmore-Dobbyn, are more common.

For Blackmore-Dobbyn, as well as for the many people who have suffered brain injuries and are of low resources, the costly and long-lasting treatments that are often required to fully recover aren't feasible. For those who live in the United States with no health insurance, there's no any hope of getting this level of care.

Within the United Kingdom, with the National Health Service, possible delays in diagnosis and treatment are not uncommon.

Blackmore-Dobbyn Blackmore-Dobbyn, a New York chef, was assaulted on the street, repeatedly punched across the forehead, choked and then had his head hit the pavement. The traumas could be enough to trigger MTBI.

In an article written for The Huffington Post in November 2011 "Why Gabby Giffords' Recovery Is Not a Miracle," Blackmore-Dobbyn said that he is not apprehensive about the care that the congresswoman was lucky enough to get.

Blackmore-Dobbyn, however lost his job and no one else to turn to for support other than his wife. "I no longer function at the same level due to chronic anxiety, permanent short-term memory impairment and a diminished capacity for multi-tasking, all of which are so vitally important in the work of a restaurant kitchen," Blackmore-Dobbyn wrote.

"I currently am employed in a lower capacity and earn less in my lifetime due to this. In the end I was financially professional, as well as emotionally destroyed. I'm not sure if this could have been different if I had have had access to rehabilitation specialists. I wish I had the choice."

Blackmore-Dobbyn suffered physical assault however he could have equally easily been involved in an auto accident or fallen from a ladder, or injured multiple times while playing contact sports, and suffered similar long-term effects. This is what the overwhelming majority of people don't know about the significance of "mild" traumatic brain injury.

Where MTBI is Concerned, Language is Deceiving

Words can be confusing. When it comes to brain injuries phrases such as "minimal", "moderate" as well as "mild" are widely misconstrued. The first trauma could appear to be "mild." The person isn't likely to lose consciousness or experience any loss of consciousness, and may have no obvious signs or symptoms for a long time, or even for days. This is because of the sly nature of this kind in brain injury.

There's likely to be there is nothing "mild" about the consequences of the injury. Indeed one of the biggest obstacles to diagnosing MTBI is the response of the patient.

If they're denial of the injury or are aware of it and avoiding their issues in fear of being rejected or even criticism It is more typical for MTBI sufferers not to seek treatment. There's a possibility that the person doesn't think that a brain injury is an option. They just know something isn't quite right. In each of these scenarios, the person is attempting to manage by themselves, even until they reach self-isolation , or self-medicating.

They are aware that they're suffering from headaches and difficulty staying focused, they feel stressed or angry or cannot endure bright lights or loud sounds, but they're not looking injured. Perhaps they "got their bell rung" while playing football, or perhaps they were involved in a collision. It's nothing to get rid of you think? Wrong.

How can MTBI diagnosed?

The ability to accurately diagnose MTBI is a major obstacle which prevents the proper treatment. The criteria that were developed in the Centres for Disease Control in the United States are as follows:

Injury to the head caused by an acceleration, blunt force, or acceleration or.

Any of the following needs to be present within the first hour following the event or during the duration of surveillance.

- Self-reported or observed impaired awareness, disorientation, or temporary confusion.

Amnesia that was self-reported or observed during the time of incident.

There are signs that suggest neurological or neuropsychological dysfunction.

The symptoms could be, but aren't restricted to:

- seizures

Lethargy, irritability and vomiting (especially in infants and young children)

headaches, dizziness, fatigue, and poor focus (in the older and more mature children as well as adults)

The CDC definition however calls for "loss of consciousness or altered consciousness" lasting at least 30 minutes for these symptoms to indicate MTBI.

The Brain Injury Association of America on its website with information about "Mild Brain Injury and Concussion" is not happy with this approach, stating:

"The definition is focused on the injury itself or symptoms, not on the possible outcomes. For many , there difficulties in obtaining correct diagnosis and proper treatment particularly in the absence of a evident or documented impairment of the brain. There doesn't need to be an absence of consciousness in order in order for a brain injury to be diagnosed."

The issue of making accurate diagnoses will be addressed more in depth within Chapter 3: Diagnosing Mild and moderate brain Trauma But this is certainly an aspect that is a part of MTBI treatments that are in need of improvement and constant application.

The Definition of MTBI and Its Major Causes

It is important to note that the definitions of MTBI is more specific that the diagnosis criteria. In the event of an external force which is either deliberate or accidental the brain's function takes place. This could result from an impact, or a "blast" force, or the rapid acceleration or acceleration of the head.

A penetrating injury isn't in the present and there could not be any loss of consciousness. The full extent of damage may not be readily evident and will be revealed as time passes.

The main factors that cause MTBI within the United States:

The rate of decline is 35.2 percent (in the U.S.)

Falls are responsible for 50% of brain injuries suffered by children aged 0-14 years old, and 61% in those aged 65 and over.

- traffic or motor vehicle accidents 17 percent

- struck by or against incidents 16.5 percent

These incidents include collisions against a fixed or moving object. They are the second most common causes of brain injuries among children aged 0-14 (in 25 percent of instances.)

- assaults 10 10%

Assaults are responsible for 2.9 percent of brain injuries for children aged 0-14 and one percent of injuries among adults who are 65 or older.

Other 21 percent

Within the United States, 18% of brain injuries are seen among children 0-4 and around 22% of these occurring for adults aged 75 or older. For 59% instances those who suffer from brain injuries are males.

Around 1.7 million residents in U.S. suffer some type of brain injury each year. Of these, more than 475,000 of them are children.

Every year, more 50 000 people die as a result of brain injuries.

It is believed at 3.1 million American citizens have a life-long disability due to brain injuries.

The CDC estimates the medical expenses and lost productivity each year due for brain injuries in excess of $76.3 billion.

(See: "What Are the Leading Causes of TBI?" The Centers for Disease Control http://www.cdc.gov/traumaticbraininjury/causes.html Accessed June 2013.)

In Europe the most common reasons for MTBI are:

Motor vehicle accidents 50 percent

This number includes automobiles, trucks, motorcycles bicycles, pedestrian injuries.

Falls, within the age group of 65+

Transport-related injuries for the 65 and younger age group

Sports-related accidents (300,000 annually)

About 20 000 are the result of the ice-skating and skiing as well as other winter sports.

Around one million injuries to the head each year across Europe and around 135,000 patients being admitted to hospitals to receive treatment.

There is a consensus that in Europe the population is 500,000 individuals between the ages of 16 and 74 with permanent disabilities caused by brain injuries.

In the case of injuries reported annually the majority of them of them are classified as mild.

Men are three times more likely an injury to the brain, and the aged 15 to 25 5 times as likely.

(See: "Brain Injury Facts," International Brain Injury Association, http://www.internationalbrain.org/brain-injury-facts/ - Accessed June 2013.)

Difficulty in Detecting MTBI

Brain injuries can be classified as diffuse or focal. A brain injury that is focal occurs at a specific location and is often related to an exact injury that involves the head being struck or hit with an object.

A diffuse brain injury is more prevalent and usually the cause of the skull increasing or slowing down. The head doesn't necessarily touch anything.

MTBI can also be due to a deficiency of oxygen in various situations that involve cerebral anoxia or hypoxia.

Cerebral Anoxia and Cerebral Hypoxia

Hypoxia and anoxia are two terms used to describe the absence of oxygen to the brain. The terms are often utilized in conjunction. In reality, the terms are used to define degrees of deprivation. Anoxia is the term used to describe damage that result from a complete deficiency of oxygen in the brain. Hypoxia refers to a reduced or insufficient quantity of oxygen that is delivered to the brain.

Causes of Anoxic or Hypoxic Brain Trauma

Anoxic brain injuries and hypoxic brain injuries can result from brain trauma that is the result of carbon monoxide poisoning drowning intoxication, suffocation, choking head trauma, bleeding that is severe or a drops in blood pressure, or stroke.

Anaesthesia mistakes as well as other surgical errors can also be the cause of decreased blood flow to the brain, which results in brain damage due to oxic. Damage to the brain caused by a deficiency of oxygen is also observed in infants, usually because of medical errors or complications that occurred during the birth of the infant.

Signs and Symptoms of Cerebral Anoxia or Hypoxia

The symptoms of brain injury due to oxygen deprivation are dependent on the severity and amount of time the brain is deprived of oxygen.

Most often, people will be distracted, have poor judgement, and may suffer from memory loss and weak motor coordination.

If the deficiency of oxygenation to the brain continues for more than a few minutes, the brain cells begin to die, leading to irreparable brain injury, comas seizures, or even death.

Treatment for Anoxia and Hypoxia

The treatment of hypoxia and anoxia is to improve an individual's blood pressure as well as the flow of oxygen into the brain. It could also involve blood transfusions, the administration of oxygen, as well as medication to reduce seizures.

Brain Damage Following Cerebral Anoxia or Hypoxia

The severity of brain damage is determined by duration for which your brain has been deprived of oxygen. It is aware that it only takes some minutes of deprivation of oxygen for brain cells to start to end up dying.

In the longer that the brain is deprived of oxygen that it needs The greater the chance of damage to the brain or the greater likelihood of coma and death. People who are recovering from the loss of oxygen typically experience memories that are lost and personality changes, behavioral changes, hallucinations, amnesia and muscle injuries.

In the event that there is a significant loss of oxygen levels in the brain, it is impaired, leading to the condition of coma. Since brain damage is very serious, the likelihood of a successful recovery is extremely slim.

The Mechanics of a MTBI

The brain is far less solid than many think. The consistency is closer to gelatine, with the whole structure being suspended in cerebrol-spinal fluid. While the bony skull shields your brain from injury, it could be a an element of the mechanism that can harm it.

When the head is exposed to a violent and sudden attack or motion, speeding up or slowing down the brain, it will impact the uneven, rough interior of skull.

The motion as well as the collision can cause the nerve cells, also known as axons, that resemble threads, stretch and strain.

Similar to when the neck experiences rapid and violent turning the twisting motion can cause the same effect. In both instances the location of neurons changes and neural cells may even be damaged.

The two motions -- rotation and impact are both forms of concussion.

The imbalance of the Axons, along with the swelling, seriously disrupts the brain's neuronal circuits, resulting in serious cognitive problems and physical damage.

More nefarious, however is the impact on the ability of cells to make the structural proteins that allow them to keep their dimensions.

This loss of axon elasticity could be the reason for the inconsistently delayed symptoms with MTBI cases.

In recovery, cells attempt to restore their equilibrium, however this could require adjustments to the original alignments or creating new alignments to adjust.

If this occurs repeatedly such as the case of repeated concussions the process of restructuring is longer every time, and each version will be less efficient than preceding one. 20 percent of those who sustain even one concussion do not fully recover.

Chapter 20: Brain Injury Measurement

In the case of a head injury, certain types of neuroimaging are utilized to evaluate the damage. However , neither CT scans or MRI scans will reveal the type of damage that is present in an MTBI as the damage can be felt in the brain's "white matter" or neuron connections.

Advances in Imaging Technology

New imaging techniques have demonstrated promise in the field in MTBI diagnosis, however the tests are costly and are not widely accessible.

These comprise:

- Positron Emission Tomography (PET)

- Single Photon Emission Computerized Tomography (SPECT)

- Functional Magnetic Resonance Imaging (fMRI)

- Diffuse Tensor Imaging (DTI)

Be aware that your health insurance might not cover certain tests that are considered "non-standard."

Neuropsychological Assessment Remains the Standard

In the majority of instances, MTBI is identified by studying the symptoms experienced by the patient. It involves testing to determine the brain's function in various areas which include, but are not only:

Attention span

- Memory

Concentration

Language

- Mathematical reasoning

- spatial perception

Abstract and Organization Thinking

- Problem solving

- social judgement

Motor skills

- Sensory awareness

General psychological adjustment

A neuropsychological examination is typically the initial step for the rehabilitation program. It assists medical professionals in determining the areas of the brain that are damaged and also the ones that are functioning normally.

Scales and Measurement of Functioning

In order to determine the extent the severity of brain injuries as well as the speed of recovery, various measurements scales are utilized.

Disability Rating Scale (DRS)

This measure was designed by working with adults and juveniles who suffer from moderate to severe levels of brain damage. The scale was developed within an inpatient rehabilitation facility to monitor patients ' progress from "coma to community."

The scale ranges from zero to 29 with 0 representing not functionally impaired while 29 is in a vegetative state. For it to be considered "reliable," the score must be determined when the patient isn't anesthetized, recovering from surgery anaesthesia, or under the influence of drugs that alter mind or following the occurrence of seizures.

The results are hoped to provide a complete picture of physical and cognitive impairment or impairment.

Functional Independent Measure (FIM)

This scale provides a measure of an individual's capacity to be able to work independently when performing daily living tasks, including self-care, managing elimination requirements, mobility (including transfers) as well as communication as well as social interaction.

The scale ranges between 1 and 7, 7 being total dependence, and 7 indicating complete independence.

Functional Assessment Measure (FAM)

The test was created to complement the Functional Independent Measure that is designed to specifically examine cognitive, behavioural communicative, and social functioning test.

The FAM is comprised of 12 items, which when combined with the 18 items in the FIM create a scale of 30 points.

(Note that a more specific version FAM is utilized by clinicians in the United Kingdom that is regarded as more objective by British health professionals.)

Glasgow Coma Scale

The rating scale is designed to measure the initial degree of brain injury in the emergency room. Patients are evaluated on their verbal, motor and eye responses.

Three is a sign of severe neurological impairment while 15 indicates normal or "near" normal.

Rancho Los Amigos (Original)

The scale is utilized in rehabilitation programs to evaluate the patterns and stages of recovery from brain injuries in terms of cognitive functioning. The scale is described as follows:

Level 1 - No Response

The sound, sight, or movement does not provoke a response by the individual. The patient must be assisted in every way.

Level 2 - Generalized Response

The sound, sight, or movement can trigger slow irregular, but frequently delayed responses. These may be accompanied by sweating, chewing rapid breathing, moaning movements, or changes of blood pressure. Complete assistance is needed.

Level 3 - Localized Response

The patient awakes at various times throughout the day. They can react to stimuli, but it is slow and infrequently.

Family and friends will be evident There will be the ability to follow simple instructions as well as respond inconsistently and non-verbally "yes" and "no" questions. The complete assistance of the caregiver is required.

Level 4 - Confused and Agitated

The patient is terrified and confused without understanding what's happening. If uncontrolled, overreactions to stimuli could lead to self-harm.

There will be a high concentration on the most essential needs, a failure to focus or follow instructions, and irregular recognition of friends and family. Maximum assistance is needed.

Level 5 - Confused and Inappropriate

The patient is capable of paying attention for a short period however, they will become confused and may have trouble comprehending his surroundings. They may not be aware of the time or the location of their body or where they are. They will also not be able complete basic daily tasks with no clear instructions.

Long-term memory will be more efficient than short-term memory, and sensory overload is the issue. Filling in gaps with assumptions (confabulation) is normal. Maximum assistance is required.

Level 6 - Confused and Appropriate

Cognitive and memory problems could be present, but the patient will be able recall the key details of conversations, even if there aren't precise details.

There is a possibility to follow a schedule with assistance , and there will be a sense that the date of each month is also a the year in the absence of a specific date.

Attention span is approximately 30 minutes without distracting sources of stimulation. Self-care can be managed, and there will be a sense that there is an injury, however it is more in terms of physical impairment rather than cognitive impairment.

There is a tendency to connect problems with being in a hospital and the belief that everything will be okay once they are home. It is essential to receive moderate assistance.

Level 7 - Automatic and Appropriate

Patients with these conditions can adhere to the prescribed schedule and keep up with regular self-care, without assistance. They might have difficulty creating plans, starting, and completing tasks.

Concentration is affected in stressful or distracting situations as well as there is an insufficient understanding of how issues with memory and cognition may make it difficult to return to former life or work conditions. A minimal amount of assistance to maintain everyday living skills is needed.

Level 8 - Purposeful and Appropriate

The patients are aware that they struggle with memory and thinking and will be actively developing strategies for compensating. They'll become more flexible, and inclined to be evaluated however their development is likely to be lower rate, which could result in sensory overload when faced by difficulties.

In new situations, poor judgment is a concern and guidance when making decisions can help. The degree of cognitive impairment that these patients experience might not be apparent to those who did not have any idea of their injuries. Assistance from a stand-by person is the best option in these situations.

Rancho Los Amigos (Revised)

The new version of this scale has the original 8 levels , and it adds two more levels:

Level 9 - Purposeful, Appropriate: Stand-By Assistance on Request

The patients can independently switch between different tasks, and maintain their attention and accuracy for upto two hours at the same time. Memory devices that aid in planning and tasks lists can be helpful however, the patient can start and complete the necessary steps to complete tasks related to household and work.

Patient is conscious and is aware of their disability and limitations. They think about the implications of their choices and evaluate their capabilities.

They might struggle with depression and irritability, and may be prone to a low tolerance for anger, however they can self-monitor for the appropriateness.

Level 10 - Purposeful, Appropriate: Modified Independent

They are able to are able to handle multiple tasks however, they will require periodic breaks. They are able to independently acquire memory aid devices and are able to independently begin projects at home and at work. They anticipate issues related to their limitations and adjust in a manner that is appropriate.

They are able to be aware of and respond to the needs and feelings of others and react to them in a manner that is appropriate. A period of depression or irritability may be present, as well as moderate levels of anger. Their behavior in social situations is constant and appropriate.

A Caution Regarding Cognitive Testing

In all cognitive tests is to be aware that results could differ widely from person to person. The variance in results could result from the context where the test is being administered or it could be the result of something that has been "stuck" in the person's memory.

In this way, patients with Alzheimer's disease are capable attaining perfect scores on their cognitive tests during the initial stages of the disease, even if their behavioral symptoms are evident.

The reason is that they simply kept, for no apparent reason, the information needed for answering the test questions.

Every cognitive test result regardless of the extent that a brain has been injured, need to be evaluated with a certain amount of caution and weighed closely against functional abilities.

Emerging Awareness of MTBI

Due to the conflicts that have raged in Iraq and Afghanistan and Afghanistan, brain trauma has been brought to the forefront of people's consciousness. Brain injuries that are severe constitute one of the "signature" wound of these conflict, and this has led to major improvement in the treatment process and long-term outlook for recovery success.

Awareness of the consequences of MTBI however, and in particular the cumulative effects of multiple injuries such as concussions has taken longer to emerge both in medical circles and within the general populace.

The consequences of these can be complex psychological and emotional responses to a trauma such as the post-traumatic stress disorder. The effects of the trauma and the emotional consequences that can last for a long time from the trauma that resulted from the incident, makes the diagnosis more challenging.

Since 2000, there were 220,430 instances in the form of TBI (Traumatic brain injury) within U.S. servicemen. Of these 60 to 80% were MTBIs which wasn't fully brought into the public eye until 2007 and wasn't reported the line commandants until the year 2009. In that year, officers were aware of the possibility that MTBI could lead to:

- diminished marksmanship

- slow response times

- lower concentration

Based on those results, the criteria used to send soldiers back to combat environments was rethought and changed.

Kathy Helmick, Deputy Director of the Defence Centres of Excellence, speaking at the 4th Annual Trauma Spectrum Conference in December of 2011 was mentioned in an article by U.S. Medicine, saying "Mild TBI remains little understood and hard to diagnose."

"There's a dire necessity to find an objective marker for concussion," Helmick declared. "We have been very much challenged and prompted by Congress to find this objective marker beyond the clinical judgment."

Potential avenues to better diagnose comprise measurements of:

Papillary response, visual tracking

- - saliva, serum, and biomarkers of the skin

- Diffuse Tensor Imaging

Electrophysiological parameters

Today, however doctors are in the majority of cases simply talking with their patients and attempt to come up with a diagnosis decision by the information they receive.

One of the biggest hurdles in finding out MTBI is the patient. A lot of them hide their issues and seek ways to overcome the cognitive impairments they face or doesn't know what's the issue.

Because many of the signs of MTBI are delaying and the effects of cumulative MTBI aren't fully recognized, it is not known how many patients suffer from this condition on their own and in isolation.

Case Study: Falling - The Most Common Cause of MTBI

On the 16th of June, 2011, Heather Marsh, DCoE Strategic Communications published an article in the Defence Centres of Excellence for Psychological Health and Traumatic Brain Injury (DCoE) which was titled "My Discovery of Mild Traumatic Brain Injury," in which she discusses her own "cluelessness" of the topic.

In March of 2011, Marsh fell, face forward on the floor which needed a trip into the emergency room and five stitches. She returned home and realized that the scratched up ego of her was one of the worst parts of the entire incident.

In the course of around ten days, she felt frightened feelings of disorientation and helplessness. Marsh talked to her DCoE colleagues among them one who was the former neurology chief and was able to realize she had suffered an injury to her head called a concussion.

Regardless of the place she worked and with whom she worked, Marsh didn't know that falls are the most common reason for mild traumatic brain injuries (MTBI).

Marsh suffered from a range of symptoms, such as a feeling of fearful anxiety just from looking at the sunlight glinting through the trees during an evening drive. "I felt a sudden rush of panic as if I was intoxicated," she wrote. "I felt disoriented and blinded all at once."

Luckily, she was able get off to on the other side to recover herself for the journey to home. The incident made her think whether returning American veterans cope with the intense sensory overload due to numerous MTBIs that they have sustained during combat.

Marsh's symptoms of concussion resolving gradually however, she emerged from her experience with MTBI aware that no one is able to explain what's simply "wrong."

Marsh gained by working with experts that helped her comprehend the damage that was occurring to her body. Otherwise she could remain silent and scared without any concrete details about the injury.

Chapter 21: Diagnosing Minimal And Moderate Brain Trauma

As with other medical conditions there isn't a perfect biomarker that can be used to identify a traumatic brain injury on any level. A biomarker is an identifiable physical characteristic that is used to assess or determine the progression or effects of a disorder or disease.

To be considered "perfect," a biomarker for TBI must meet five very specific requirements:

Indicate the nature of the injury on the brain.

- - Appear in some biological fluid, possibly blood, within the first hour of the trauma that caused the TBI.

Connectivity with measures derived from neuroimages as well as scores for neurological disorders.

Predict the course of the that will result from the TBI.

Allow for monitoring of follow-up and adjustments to therapies and medicines.

The absence of the "perfect" biomarker, however it does not mean that researchers haven't made important progress in the development of quantifiable tests to diagnose brain trauma.

The Evolution of Blood-Based Diagnostics for TBI

In the past five years, researchers have tried to create the measurement of cell blood-borne proteins secreted proteins, peptides and peptides as well as proteolytic fragments (created through the breakdown of protein.) The initial clinical trials showed poor performance, and failed to meet the five main specifications.

In 2011 however, a research study, published in Annals of Emergency Medicine, found that there was an increase in acidic proteins in blood of patients suffering from TBI. The researchers suggested that testing for the protein that is administered within the first four hours after the injury's initial occurrence could give an accurate assessment of the degree of head trauma that is present.

The most reliable indication which has emerged since then has been the serum protein S100B which is found usually exclusively in the brain. If it's found inside the bloodstream it means that the brain-blood barrier has been damaged and a brain injury may have been sustained, even though there are no signs or symptoms.

The blood-brain-brain barrier acts as a constantly-changing, secure barrier, which separates the brain and central nervous system, from the harmful substances that circulate through the system of circulation.

The presence of a serum protein alone might indicate the presence of brain trauma, however the ultimate goal is what researchers in "Blood-Based Diagnostics of Traumatic Brain Injuries" (Expert Review of Molecular Diagnostics January 2011,) described as "a multimarker strategy that could be useful in refining risk stratification and for categorizing patients with TBI."

In addition the same report concluded its findings with this alarming conclusion:

"The magnitude as well as the complexity challenges that are posed by TBI are often undervalued. The current classification systems are not enough. There is no clinical method accessible to make a reliable evaluation for the degree of trauma as well as the outcome of patients with TBI particularly those with mild TBI as mild TBI patients experience only minor impairments."

Brain Injury Testing in Professional Sports

Researchers from The Cleveland Clinic and at the University of Rochester are actively researching long-term changes to the brain among professional football players.

According to studies released by the National Institute for Occupational Safety and Health in Cincinnati in Neurology (September 2012) are at a higher chance of developing neurodegenerative diseases, including but not only Parkinson's disease and Alzheimer's.

The Dr. Damir Janigro, the director of research in cerebrovascular health at Cleveland Clinic's Lerner Research Institute was quoted in Medical News Today in March 2013 "Much attention is being paid to concussions among football players and the big hits that cause them, but research shows that more common 'sub-concussive' hits appear to cause damage, too."

In the 67 footballers who participated with study Cleveland Clinic study, S100B levels increased, despite the fact that none of the participants had been diagnosed with concussions. Four of the participants were positive for a neurodegenerative disease in their measurable immune reactions based on the tests of blood.

If S100B is present in bloodstream, it triggers an autoimmune reaction. Antibodies are released and get to the brain , where they adversely affect the tissue and cause long-term brain damage.

Alongside blood tests to determine S100B concentrations, athletes had brain scans taken, and were assessed for motor control and timing of reaction, balance and memory.

About 40% of professional footballers within the United States suffer at least one concussion per year. A test called the S100B test has been shown to be an excellent measure of the severity of brain trauma. And it comes for a price of 40 dollars per PS27, in comparison to far more costly and less accurate methods such as CT scans and MRI scans.

Blood Testing for Concussion Used in Europe, Not U.S.

However the test for blood levels of S100B although extensively utilized across Europe in emergency departments as a screening procedure for concussions, have not been as widely recognized within the United States.

This sad fact is even with the high demand for more effective evaluation tools for MTBI particularly among parents of young athletes.

This increasing concern stems from the scientifically proven connection between long-term degenerative brain disorders and concussion as demonstrated by the tragic deaths of NFL players like the former San Diego Charger linebacker Junior Seau who shot himself in 2012. The autopsy revealed that he had chronic trauma encephalopathy also known as CTE which is caused by frequent head blows throughout his time playing professionally.

In an article written by Bill Pennington, "A New Way to Care for Young Brains" which was published in The New York Times on May 5, 2013 Doctor. William Meehan, co-founder of the Sports Concussion Clinic at Boston's Children's Hospital, said, "It was an entirely different story where a father of a child coming in with a sigh of relief to say, 'He's healthy; this concussion stuff is all nonsense.

But it's different now. A child is suffering from a concussion, and parents are extremely concerned about how they'll manage him when he reaches 50."

CTE can trigger the same symptoms to those of Alzheimer's, which include changes in behavior, major depressive symptoms, loss of memory and problems with the control of impulses.

At present, CTE can only be definitively diagnosed post-mortem. But it has been observed in professional athletes as well as young athletes who have attempted to commit suicide.

The issue has garnered enough attention from the United States that 47 states and the District of Columbia have now adopted the Lystedt Law. This law requires all athletes who have suffered concussions to get written permission from a doctor (often one with a background in the field of concussion treatment) before they are allowed to return to playing.

Another aspect that is more challenging to resolve the issue is the athletes themselves. In a study by researchers from Cincinnati Children's Academy only a quarter of the high school athletes who were surveyed were able to say that they wouldn't report symptoms of concussion to their coaches to allow them to return to playing. A majority of these athletes admitted to being conscious of the potential for serious injury resulting from this decision.

Emerging Picture of the Seriousness of MTBI

The study into a blood-based test procedure for MTBI has shown that repeated injuries towards the head even when absence of concussions that are diagnosed reduce the strength of the barrier between blood and brain. If the barrier is weak then brain damage at least in part is inevitable.

The full impact of such injuries might not be evident in the long run, as evidenced by the latest knowledge about CTE. Even in instances that show "complete recovery" from a concussion, your brain will not be exactly the same.

Solutions to this issue have varied from attempts to improve head protection equipment, to the increasing number of "youth concussion clinics" adjacent to major hospitals across the United States.

Recent research suggests that higher-tech, heavier helmets are not enough to reduce the danger of concussion. A study was released in July 2013, looking at 1300 high school footballers from various schools students wearing traditional helmets had the same amount of protection from concussion when compared to those who were wearing newer models.

The study's author is the researcher Dr. Timothy McGuine, research director at the University of Wisconsin Health Sports Medicine Centre in Madison stated, "The helmet technology is modern as can be. They've done an amazing job. There aren't any brain fractures during football. However,

I'm not sure the amount of padding that can be put in place to stop the brain from moving within the cranium."

(Source: "Concussion Prevention: Pass on Pricey Football Helmets, Study Suggests," MedlinePlus, 15 July 2013, http://www.nlm.nih.gov/medlineplus/news/fullstory_138698.html , accessed July 2013.)

Only in Europe However, only in Europe have doctors begun to embrace blood tests as a reliable method to determine elevated levels of protein as a sign for "mild" brain injury.

As long as these tests are not widely accepted and utilized to avoid re-injury, greater than 1.5 million concussions that happen throughout the U.S. each year, and also those that occur because of contact sports across the globe will not cease.

The process of recovering from MTBI and dealing with its effects is the costs that patients are required to bear as medical science struggles in order to fully comprehend and deal with a condition which is often described to be "mild."

Case Study: Youngest Case of Chronic Traumatic Encephalopathy on Record

In 2009, researchers from the clinical research department at the Center to Study Traumatic Encephalopathy in the Boston University School of Medicine revealed their findings of the degenerative brain disorder in the autopsy of an 18-year-old multi-sport athlete.

The name of the person was kept secret due to the wishes of his parents is the youngest individual ever identified with the brain degenerative condition.

If the boy was alive in the past, he could have suffered from early-onset dementia like that which is found in many NFL players like the former San Diego Charger linebacker Junior Seau who likely suffered an astounding 1,500 concussions over his 15-year career as a professional football player.

The Dr. Ann McKee, a neurologist and director of the brain banks at BU explained that of the thousands of post-mortem examinations they have conducted, the traumatic encephalopathy had only been found in athletes, and not in all people.

The teenager suffered multiple concussions while playing football in high school as well as other sports that involved contact, and was also a participant in contact sports for a week preceding his death. The circumstances surrounding his death were not revealed except to say that the circumstances were not a result of violent head injuries or assault.

A former Harvard soccer player, professional wrestling champion Chris Nowinski, co-director of the BU center and the author of Head Games: Football's Concussion Crisis stated, "This should be a alarm signal, particularly to parents, coaches, and league officials. We're risking the lives of more than one million children to early-onset brain damage , and we're not sure what we can do to avoid it."

Sources: Bob Hohler, "Major Breakthrough in Concussion Crisis: Researchers Find Signs of Degenerative Brain Disease in an 18-Year-Old High School Player," The Boston Globe, 27 January 2009,

http://www.boston.com/sports/other_sports /articles/2009/01/27/major_breakthrough_in _concussion_crisis/?page=full (Accessed July 2013); "Case Study: 18 Year Old High School Football Player," BU Centre for the Study of Traumatic Encephalopathy, http://www.bu.edu/cste/case-studies/18-year-old/ (Accessed July 2013).

Chapter 22: The Journey Towards Recovery

There isn't a standard schedule for recovering from brain injuries. Each instance in MTBI is as unique as the person who is suffering from the injury. Sometimes the neurons of the brain recover. Sometimes , they do not. However, recovering from MTBI isn't a quick process.

Most of the time, you'll encounter the disdain and insensitivity of people around you who think that you are beautiful. It is inevitable that you will be a victim of your own anger because you are the only one who will be conscious that you're not "fine."

The general rules and knowledge on MTBI to aid you, your family and your fellow patients, however your journey will be entirely yours.

Your Injury May Initially Be Dismissed Out of Hand

Let's suppose you're involved in a car accident. Maybe your car is hit from behind , and you're being thrown forward until your head snaps backwards.

The motion is known as coup and the coutrecoup. The brain first makes an impact when it shoots forward and strikes in the forehead of the skull. It is then injured by snapping backward and strikes the back of the skull.

The vehicle comes to a halt. There's no bleeding and you're not bleeding, however, you suffering from headache. However, generally you're glad of being alive.

Then, the paramedics arrive. You've got your name. You are aware of which fingers technology is holding. To be sure However, you have agreed to visit an emergency department.

You will receive the CT scan, or perhaps you get an MRI scan. There's no blood. You're feeling "banged up," but you're able to think. Doctor gives you two aspirins and takes you home. The doctor may or may not notify you that you've suffered an injury to your head.

If the doctor diagnoses concussion in you, his advice is likely to be to take as little as you can for the next 2 or 3 weeks until your brain has had a an opportunity to recover.

At this point it is important to reduce audio and visual stimuli in the maximum extent possible. The most important thing is to avoid all stimuli.

The next day, you awake feeling like you've been struck by the most severe case of influenza you could ever imagine. In the following few days, the symptoms become worse. You're trying to sleep often. You're sad, even grieving but are unable to describe what happened during the incident.

It is difficult to understand when you tryto figure it out, and you end up breaking down. Your spouse and your friends are supportive. They think you're upset and angry. This will pass. But it's not. You hear a ringing inside your ears. It's hard to think. You can't sleep. You might stumble, or even seek out words.

Light can cause discomfort to your eyes, and sound your ears, and so you seek out a place that is cool and peaceful and shut yourself in. A book read to pass time doesn't do the trick because after two minutes you've finished reading a book, you're not able to remember the words.

Food smells bad to you. The colors are bright. Every noise irritates your nerves. A couple of weeks pass and then the day comes where you believe you're doing better and you attempt to get yourself motivated to do something accomplished.

You decide to go to the nearby store. After an hour of pulling off your parking lot, you're circling around in circles in a haze of tears, lost and unsure of where you're at.

It takes you a whole week to come to terms with the incident then you purchase an GPS. It helps you find the best route to go around your city every day, since you're always confused and not just with directions, but for everything. Simple questions can send you into state of panic, especially when you're under pressure to respond immediately.

Afraid and embarrassed by what's going on You attempt to hide your symptoms But the stress on your brain gets too much.

Then, you short circuit. With all the information in your system, and no capacity to sort and understand the meaning of all the information it is time to acknowledge that something is extremely wrong.

While it's insane as it might be for anyone to endure that kind of emotional and physical discomfort to get their injury acknowledged as legitimate, a variations of this happen to MTBI sufferers each day.

If you do reach the point of being totally incapable of functioning, don't always think that medical experts will behave in the manner you would expect them to ought to.

It's a sad reality of MTBI that doctors are more ignorant than knowledgeable about the actual severity of the condition.

In the event of confusion from doctors that are supposed to assist you, it might be your family members and your friends who are able to recognize the issue.

The seriousness of MTBI is only recognized in the past five years, and the long-term treatment and treatment of the condition are still at an alarmingly primitive stage of development. This lack of correct medical intervention is what makes the condition even more enraged.

Brain Injuries Present in Physical Ways

Although there is no obvious bodily injuries in the case of MTBI the results of the injury will be manifest physically. If the cognitive and functional drop out were not enough there are other issues you could be dealing with:

Balance issues, including vertigo and dizziness

The stomach and nausea

- Shoulder and neck pain, as well as migraines, and pain in the scalp

Jaw grinding and clenching (day as well as at night)

- Back discomfort

- Choking and swallowing in a way that isn't even with food or saliva

It's not uncommon for an individual's prescription for glasses to change following MTBI as well as for females to experience an altered hormonal cycle.

It is an error to consider MTBI as an individual head injury since the brain is the center of all body's systems.

When there is a problem within "command central," the results are felt throughout the body. The symptoms can become regular with time, however, while they're present, they'll make you feel "crazier."

Balance Issues

The people who have experienced an MTBI might not be able to walk in with a straight line, or shut their eyes to feel the nose's end. The sudden movements could cause a flurry of nausea, or the result can be completely unpredictable and unpredictably. As long as balance issues don't get resolved, don't drive or operate any kind of machine.

It is generally recommended to move slowly and be careful not to make abrupt changes in posture, such as standing too fast from a sitting posture, or looking up abruptly. Sometimes wearing dark glasses outdoors and indoors can help because flashes of light could induce dizziness.

Vision Problems

The extreme sensitivity to light is among of the most frequently reported effects of MTBI that is then dark spots, blurred vision or regions in the field of vision which appear blurred like they're coated with thick grease.

The ability to concentrate your eyes and utilize your peripheral vision could be affected as well. Also, dark glasses aid and you should stay clear of using machines.

If the visual issues persist after a couple of weeks, consult your eye doctor. It's possible that you will require glasses, or even if you already wear glasses, then your prescription needs to be adjusted.

In a few months , you could need another eye exam as your eyes get used to normalizing however, since the consequences of vision disturbances are intense, it's best to buy glasses rather than be a part of a world you aren't able to perceive.

Hormones in Disarray

Women suffering from MTBI are likely to experience a change in the menstrual cycle. It could alter in frequency or flow, as well as duration. The hormones influence all body systems from sleeping to digestion.

The fallout of hormones can be observed within the body's immune system and it could be less effective in warding against infectious agents. Patients with MTBI may be susceptible to developing coughs and colds that can drag for months and women are particularly susceptible to yeast infections.

Sexual Dysfunction

Sexual reactions are among the most complex of bodily reactions. Different systems must work together in order for someone to feel a desire for sexual intimacy. It's not uncommon for those suffering from MTBI in losing sexual desire or to not be able to perform sexually. In essence, the brain isn't able to handle all the complex processes required.

Don't rush this stage of recovery. Sexual desire and function could come back slowly, though this aspect that you live in, just like many others, might differ after MTBI. Both you as well as your partner need patience with each other. If possible, do not let self-esteem issues create a situation that is more difficult. Regain intimacy in stages.

It is essential for members to be aware that hypersensitivity could extend to physical contact regardless of how affectionate. The feeling that once was pleasant may become uncomfortable.

They must be able to be attentive and communicate, permitting new avenues of intimacy to emerge. It is possible for each person to test their own to find out the things that work and to share their findings with their spouse.

Since sexual activity is aerobic and stamina decreases after MTBI Do not be scared by a rapid heart rate or breathlessness. Slow down and do not try alcohol for a way to "take the edge off." Alcohol is a deterrent to sexual activity even in healthy individuals however, it could cause the problem to be much worse for people with MTBI.

The other side of dysfunction or disinterest at home can be unintentional behavior or intoxication. You don't just would like it, you desire to do it constantly, and not always at the right time. This is a problem that can be the most difficult for your partner.

If you suspect that sexually inappropriate behavior is a concern, get help from an experienced counsellor. It's an incident that is temporary however, it has huge potential for humiliation and damage to relationships in the event that it is not addressed.

Getting the Help of Trauma Specialists is Imperative

Many people who are suffering with MTBI are seeking the assistance of neurotrauma cases managers speech and language life coaches, therapists and other trauma specialists. They are on the most cutting-edge of MTBI recovery techniques, understand that you can't sleep from an injury to your brain.

The therapy professionals help MTBI patients create the ideal setting for healing by finding and implementing coping strategies. They could include, but certainly not restricted to:

Recognizing the difference between staying with the work, and having to put it down. Brains aren't muscular system that can be enhanced by pushing more. Doing too much can slow the recovery process from MTBI.

It is important to carry a notebook in order to keep in mind the countless small bits of information we require to be aware of in our everyday lives. Simple as having a personal reference book could help reduce the frustration that can trigger the onset of a crisis within the course of an MTBI patients' day.

- Scheduling your day-to-day routine tasks and allowing enough time to complete them according to your current pace. The last minute only adds anxiety and stress. Plan ahead and dividing tasks can make your life more manageable and allow you to feel more at ease.

Practice rehearsing difficult situations. Therapists can provide MTBI sufferers with a safe space to practice how they react to situations that they find stressful, such as the simple question, "How are you?" Since social filters frequently diminish with brain injury the patient might struggle with the amount of information they can share and may be unable to form an appropriate, non-sensical response such as, "I'm doing better."

Finding new stress-reducing activities to relieve stress. Many people suffering from MTBI are aware that the release of endorphins during exercising are extremely helpful in reducing their levels of stress. Some people enjoy activities that provide the feeling of restoring order, such as making puzzles with jigsaws or being imaginative.

Trauma specialists also collaborate with families and friends to assist them in understanding their crucial role to play in the lives of someone recovering from MTBI. Others who are close to them must be taught how to anticipate the likely reactions and come up with appropriate reactions.

The people suffering from MTBI suffer from a significant amount of guilt over being unable to do "enough," like returning to work, and are overwhelmed by the feeling that all is not enough. It is essential for them to understand that they're not the only ones suffering since a tendency towards self-insularity is extremely strong when it comes to these kinds of cases.

Family and friends are likely to experience their fair share of stress. The loved one they have come to know and admire is not reacting and acting according to the way they are used to, and they will also be scared or anxious and possibly angered.

Exploring the Fallout of MTBI

Although it can't be stressed sufficiently enough that each case of MTBI is distinct to each person, and should be treated as such but there are common elements that can be found in various ways with this type of injury.

Disruptions in Normal Thought Patterns

We have no reason to dissect the ways we think or to delineate the various elements involved in absorbing the information and manipulating it.

It could mean anything from knowing the language spoken, to solving simple math problems at lunchtime, to determining the correct amount of tip.

Patients with MTBI However, they struggle with challenges in very specific areas of their brains that impact every aspect of their lives , which includes (but not only):

Attention!

Concentration

Memory

- Reasoning

- Planning

- understanding

Language and speech

The mechanical issues spill over into a myriad of issues that are functional, ranging including anger management and sexual dysfunction.

The Interrelated Nature of Thought

We are accustomed to the ability to effortlessly shift our attention and focus in every day life. The overload of sensory stimuli MTBI sufferers face comes directly from the lack of filters to regulate sensations such as hearing and touching.

A few people suffering from MTBI claim they are experiencing the first time that in their life they can feel your feet touching ground when they walk. Others, who've always loved summer nights, suddenly hear crickets chirping unsettlingly loud and annoying.

Two cognitive functions are at play in these scenarios. The first is attention, which is the ability to focus on the specific information that our sensory system is receiving. We can normally choose to ignore or block out certain things in favour of something else. We determine the direction in which our attention should be directed.

In certain situations it is necessary to be aware of a possible stimulus in the background, such as for instance , the noise of the baby rising up from a nap.

In times of focus, we reach an unwavering focus to acquire and retaining information. Exam preparation is an excellent illustration.

For some who suffer from MTBI it is likely that they won't be able to detect sounds of newborn getting up and reading a textbook even if they succeed it is likely that they won't remember most of the information they read.

Everyone suffers from inattention at times For instance, we might find ourselves instantly losing the identity of a person whom we've had the pleasure of meeting at a dinner event. However, someone suffering from MTBI sufferer may inquire of a waiter "How much is the check?" and not remember the exact amount for in time enough to pull the money from their wallet.

For some people is the phenomenon referred to in the field of "Swiss cheese effect," that can be seen in those with long-term memory impairments and results in incapable of consistently retrieving previous information that was learned.

Someone suffering from this kind of cognitive impairment might be able to be able to recall the time when Abraham Lincoln was president, but may not be able to provide a single bit of information on Lincoln's presidency. American Civil War over which Lincoln was the president.

In the case of these short - and long-term memory deficits, MTBI patients also find the task management challenging because their perception of time has changed and their capacity to effectively allocate their time.

They struggle to judge the amount of time needed to finish certain tasks while tracking deadlines is difficult for them.

In these and other ways executive functions are a major concern for the MTBI sufferer. How can you determine the importance of one aspect over the other? What is your method of prioritizing? Since doing two tasks simultaneously can throw a person overloaded and they lose the ability to take action since they don't have a clue where to start.

In previously determined and focused individuals, the inability of take a decisive step is frightening and a sigh of relief. In fear they turn cautious and secretive, doing whatever they can to conceal their issues from the people who surround them, particularly those they live or work. If a person is suffering from communication issues, they could be easy to feel like their entire world is falling apart.

Chapter 23: When Words Fail You

Multiple brain regions are responsible for the brain's processes that enable us to speak not only and understand the flow and ebb of conversation and remain on top of the subtleties of meaning. MTBI could cause issues with:

- Articulation

- Fluency

- Attentiveness

- Interpretation

Furthermore, if the injury affects the temporal lobe your brain, you might not be able to recognize and appropriately respond to non-verbal communication that involves eye contact, expressions of posture, gestures, and posture.

The most frequent speech problems include:

Verbal Apraxia: This disorder is akin to stuttering, and it is a sign of the speaker's inability make words upon command.

-- Dysarthria It is the inability to move the muscles required to form words and pronounce them.

Dysfluency is the technical term for stuttering. It is a kind of speech characterised by a slow stammering, and partially formed words.

Dysphasia: a loss of speech in the generation of speech, and occasionally also in understanding.

As a concomitant language issue Aphasia can be present. It is, in general an inability to comprehend and express words in their proper context. For example the patient may need to use the bathroom but then ask to go to the shop.

There are three main forms of aphasia, with distinct sub-sets.

Aphasia of the speech is caused by sentence structure spelling, grammar as well as verbal reasoning and speed of speech.

A most common type is known as Broca's Aphasia. The person is able to comprehend the message being communicated to them, however they cannot respond in a fluent manner and instead uses only single words and gestures to convey their message to be understood.

An inappropriate choice of words or grammar mismatch is known as "neologism," and "anomia" is the inability of correctly naming the familiar objects.

Other variants are dysnomia (groping for words) as well as fluent (talking quickly with no meaningful content) as well as conductivity (halting speech) and persistent (uncontrolled repeating).

Receptive aphasia means difficulties with reading and interpreting both spoken and written language.

It is normal to speak however, when people speak to you, it's like you're speaking an entirely different language. If you're able to be able to comprehend a small portion of what's being spoken, you will encounter so many gaps that you're not able to react.

Other possible forms are paraphasia (the use of words that are partial) and analexia (an difficulty reading).

Mixed aphasia combines two issues with language comprehension , and expression.

Dealing with Speech and Language Problems

In the majority of instances of MTBI problems with articulation, speech and stuttering go away by themselves in 3 or less months and language impairments diminishing or improving with time, typically with the assistance of a certified speech therapist.

Therapists know how to assist you to retrain the speech centers in your brain. Additionally, they can monitor your progressand adjust methods in accordance with your progress. This could require working with a psychotherapist or psychologist to alleviate the natural and normal frustration that comes with these kinds of issues.

A few things you can try to do to help better with speech and language difficulties include (but aren't restricted to):

- Taking conscious efforts to relax by deep breathing, which can help slow down stammering.

Have important conversations and meetings in a relaxed and calm environment, that is free of distractions, which will increase your ability to understand the message and respond accordingly.

- Learning how to picture the word you would like to use as if it was on a chalkboard within your head. This will allow you to choose an appropriate word that can be said.

Create pre-planned signals with loved ones so that you be aware when you're headed off into an off-topic conversation.

Don't hide your issues. This will only add to your frustration and embarrassment.

If you've got an inclination to speak up, stop this for now. When those with MTBI are in stressful situations, they can both become angry and become less able to communicate. This is one recipe for anger!

Find ways to be creative as you practice your communication abilities. You can turn off the sound on your TV and check how you interpret the actions of characters by their expressions and other non-verbal signals.

Write down your thoughts in a journal or experiment with drawing to convey what you're thinking and feeling, while your communication skills are growing.

Although it is difficult to comprehend how frustrating this stage of your recovery might be, keep in mind that this is only a temporary stage. If you can, take a look at your own mistakes that you've made with a pinch of humor.

Anchorman Bob Woodward, during an interview, recalled the day the couple waited for long hours for an repairman for cable TV who was part of the corporation Viacom. With a sense of frustration and anger, Woodward exclaimed, "When will that Viagra man get here!"

A Broader Pattern of Symptoms

Other signs MTBI patients experience may include:

The fatigue can be crushing and cause a fatigue, particularly during the first few weeks following the injury.

Personality and behavioural changes typically are associated with controlling impulses and anger.

Post-traumatic stress disorder is characterized by reliving the experiences of the incident or having negative reactions to similar situations.

- Amnesia often relating to the event or the period immediately between the event and the time immediately following it.

Fear and anxiety which could cause agoraphobia, anxiety about leaving home.

depression, mood swings and anger, which make social interactions difficult.

Sexual dysfunctions can be emotional and/or physical in the sense that it is.

Obsessive-compulsive behavior as a means to "manage" your condition.

Sometimes , people with MTBI experience mood swings so severe that they can be classified as manic depressive.

A Word About Fatigue

It is essential to comprehend the physical aspects of fatigue and how it relates to energy that is comprised of emotional, physical and cognitive components along with your "reserves." Listen to your inner voice!

When you're exhausted you should stop and take breaks. It's not something to be embarrassed about. The fatigue could last throughout your life following MTBI.

Everyone Wants the Impossible, an Exact Prognosis

Due to the individual nature of each case of MTBI giving broad estimates of an exact diagnosis is not feasible nor reasonable. It is not possible to say that every patient will be in X condition within X amount of weeks is not a realistic scenario in these situations.

The conventional wisdom of medical science is that patients who suffer concussions recover within the space of a few weeks. It is possible the sense that any residual effects from the concussion can be considered minimal to not be noticeable as to their effect on the person's daily life.

The most significant factor that can be attributed to concussion cases is the absence or presence of the possibility of re-injury. In the case of repeated concussions each one causes it more difficult for the brain to heal itself, and the deficits get more evident.

In the most severe or numerous instances of MTBI Some patients could be unable to work for a long time and then achieve a full functional recovery.

In all instances of brain injuries generally, it is believed that the longest-term window of chance of healing is about 2-3 years. If the function is recovered, it will be restored within that time.

More and more, research suggests that the likelihood of recovery MTBI is contingent on a variety of variables, including the age.

A study published in the month of July by research scientists from the University of Oregon and the University of British Columbia showed the ongoing disruption of executive function in teenagers suffering from concussions for two months following the injury.

It is more than twice the duration of young adults. In this group cognitive function is expected to improve between about two weeks or a month.

Similar research that was conducted in 2012 revealed persistent neuropsychological problems in adolescents who had suffered concussions for at least six months following the incident.

The authors suggested a higher risk of concussion in adolescents because of the rapid development of the frontal region of the brain in this stage of life.

(Source: Lindsay Barton, "Effects of Concussion on Higher Cognitive Function Persist In Teens, Study Says," Moms Team, 5 June 2013, http://www.momsteam.com/health-safety/effects-concussion-higher-cognitive-function-persist-in-teens-study-says , accessed July 2013.)

In actual fact, it is much simpler to assign milestones to cases of traumatic brain injury than it is to cases of MTBI due to the fact that they are more individualized and difficult to determine.

At some moment, patients who've worked for months experiencing little improvement may need to consider the limitations of recovery that be like for them.

They might only be able to return to their work in a modified method, or never be able to go back to their previous work.

Their perception of their personal lives is changed by an injury that medical science has a tendency to characterize it as "mild."

For certain MTBI sufferers, they could endure the rest of their life struggling with memory problems and problem-solving thinking in deductive ways, tension emotional control, cognitive fatigue depression, anger, and anxiety. They'll certainly create an entirely new "normal," but it won't be the same as their old "normal."

Accepting the "new normal" is a vital aspect of recovery. If you don't, you'll always fighting an internal fight that will hinder your from getting over depression and problems with self-esteem.

Chapter 24 : Finding What Works

The most difficult thing that MTBI sufferers must take is accepting that their brains have been damaged and they are now dealing with the consequences of the damage for the rest of their lives.

A word such as "acceptance" can be both easy and boring without acknowledgment of the size of the changes that we're talking about. Anyone suffering from MTBI is required to at least accept the necessity of learning and monitoring their performance on tasks that were previously easy and automatic that they didn't require any thought.

Most of these roles can be described as "executive" in nature because they are essential to the everyday activities of our lives. Becoming aware of each days of the week and month does more than only help you to keep track of the calendar it's also a part in arranging your day and making your payments, meeting deadlines for work, and even getting a book returned to the library in time.

Processing Speed Batters the Self-Esteem

If a person is experiencing an impairment in their ability to comprehend and react to information, the resulting degree of anger is severe and can affect self-esteem. The world is moving at a rapid pace! You're not able to keep up and it's easy to think that you're "stupid" (and quite often to get angry because you feel horrible both physically as well as emotionally.)

It is crucial to let yourself off the hook. You're being afflicted by a brain trauma which is less defined by a visible injury but more as it is a disturbance in the metabolism of the brain.

The brain has experienced twisting, shearing, and stretching forces that have made it slack. The cells aren't functioning in the way they normally do.

Brain injuries are not an indicator of your intelligence. The idea that it is the case is the

179

same sense as declaring, "He has a broken leg so he was never a good runner."

It is important to be sure to follow your "logic" to the next step. "He" may well be an outstanding athlete, but since the leg he injured was broken it is unlikely that he will perform the same way in the future.

In the aftermath of an MTBI you might not be thinking the identical way however, you will be thinking efficiently and effectively by adjusting your thinking to new patterns that you develop to accommodate your new perception of the world.

The Effects of Slower Processing

The most frequent signs of slow processing speed are:

- The inability to focus on multiple thoughts at a single time.

- Being lost in an argument.

- Not "getting" jokes.

- Unable to keep track of plots.

Then you forget why you entered the room.

- Letting your sentences go unfinished.

Inability to recognize non-verbal signals.

Another serious problem is the inability to determine the impact of an act. The directions for a frozen meal could say, "Cook in a 450 degree F oven for 30 minutes." The instructions do not state, "Take the dinner out of the cardboard box and then put the tray in a 450 degree F oven."

A person suffering from MTBI might not catch this and throw all of the box in the oven, not realizing that the cardboard might catch the fire.

Overall Coping Mechanisms

In collaboration with rehabilitation specialists with whom you can develop individual methods of coping for your particular problems. However, there are various general-purpose techniques that can be used to lessen the cascading and interlocking consequences of MTBI.

Managing Your Environment

Overwhelmed by stimuli is a major obstacle MTBI patients have to face on a daily basis. When you are trying to get back control of your executive thoughts, creating an environment where you are able to focus is vital - both at home as well as at work.

Making adjustments to your surroundings can be as simple as switching off the TV as you pay the bills or requesting your boss to shift your desk away from an overcrowded cluster of cubicles to an area with less distractions.

Don't be afraid to request the necessary accommodations to be able to work. You are entitled to legal rights when working. The United States, people with MTBI are protected under The Americans with Disabilities Act and those living in the United Kingdom are covered by the Equality Act 2010.

If you are able to discuss your concerns with your employer, and then explain the necessity for your workplace to be modified The compliance with the request is legally required.

Seek Out Quiet Time

If you're working or at home be aware of the importance of quiet time to restore your balance and focusing. If you start to be overwhelmed, your organization skills will decrease rapidly and you might start to feel overwhelmed and panic.

In these moments it is important to go to a quiet area so that you can relax and take a break. But don't only reserve quiet moments for emergencies. Make use of quiet times throughout the daytime to avoid becoming overwhelmed.

Take a stroll in the park at lunchtime, or sit for a couple of minutes in a library or church or simply listen to a soothing tune on your headphones. "Time outs" prevent your brain from overloading and then closing down.

This could mean taking an afternoon nap whenever you feel you require one. The exhaustion of working at a high level of concentration and keep on track is often exhausting.

The more tired you get more exhausted, the less able you are to control your emotional responses. An "power nap" can work miracles when it comes to "rebooting" your brain.

www.ingramcontent.com/pod-product-compliance
Lightning Source LLC
Chambersburg PA
CBHW062139020426
42335CB00013B/1266